The Real Food Dietitians

the real food table

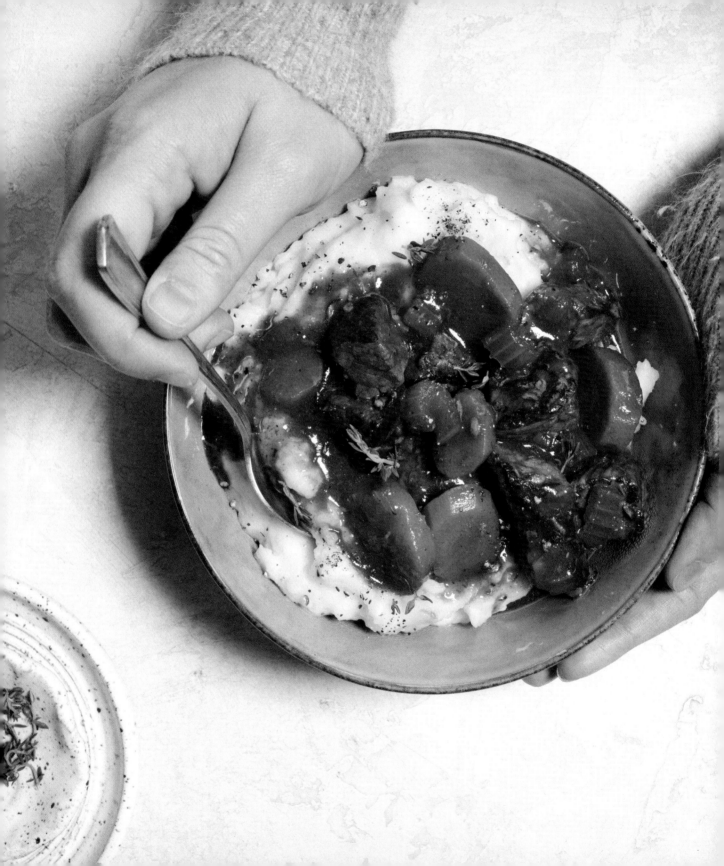

The Real Food Dietitians

the real food table

100 Easy and Delicious Mostly Gluten-Free, Grain-Free
and Dairy-Free Recipes for Every Day

Jessica Beacom, RDN, and Stacie Hassing, RDN, LD
Photography by Eliesa Johnson

Simon Element
New York   London   Toronto   Sydney   New Delhi

SIMON
ELEMENT

An Imprint of Simon & Schuster, Inc.
1230 Avenue of the Americas
New York, NY 10020

First Simon Element paperback edition March 2023

SIMON ELEMENT and colophon are trademarks of Simon & Schuster, Inc.

For information about special discounts for bulk purchases, please contact Simon &
Schuster Special Sales at 1-866-506-1949 or business@simonandschuster.com.

The Simon & Schuster Speakers Bureau can bring authors to your live event. For
more information or to book an event, contact the Simon & Schuster Speakers
Bureau at 1-866-248-3049 or visit our website at www.simonspeakers.com.

Interior design by Ruth Lee-Mui

Photography Copyright © 2022 by Eliesa Johnson

Food styling by Diana Scanlon
Prop styling by Jess Larson

Manufactured in China

1   3   5   7   9   10   8   6   4   2

Library of Congress Cataloging-in-Publication Data has been applied for.

ISBN 978-1-9821-7835-2
ISBN 978-1-6680-1504-9 (pbk)
ISBN 978-1-9821-7836-9 (ebook)

To our Real Food community:

This cookbook would have not been made possible without your continuous support and dedication to the brand. We couldn't be more excited to have an even bigger role in your kitchen for years to come, whether you're cooking from this book, finding new recipes on the website, or engaging with us and fellow community members on social media. Thank you for believing in us, and a big welcome to our Real Food Table, where there's something delicious for everyone!

contents

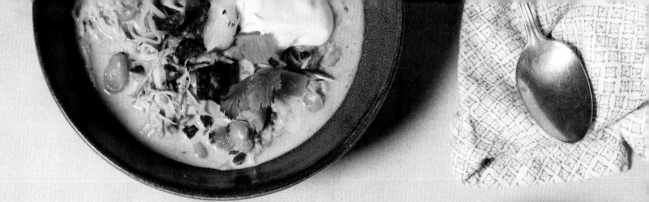

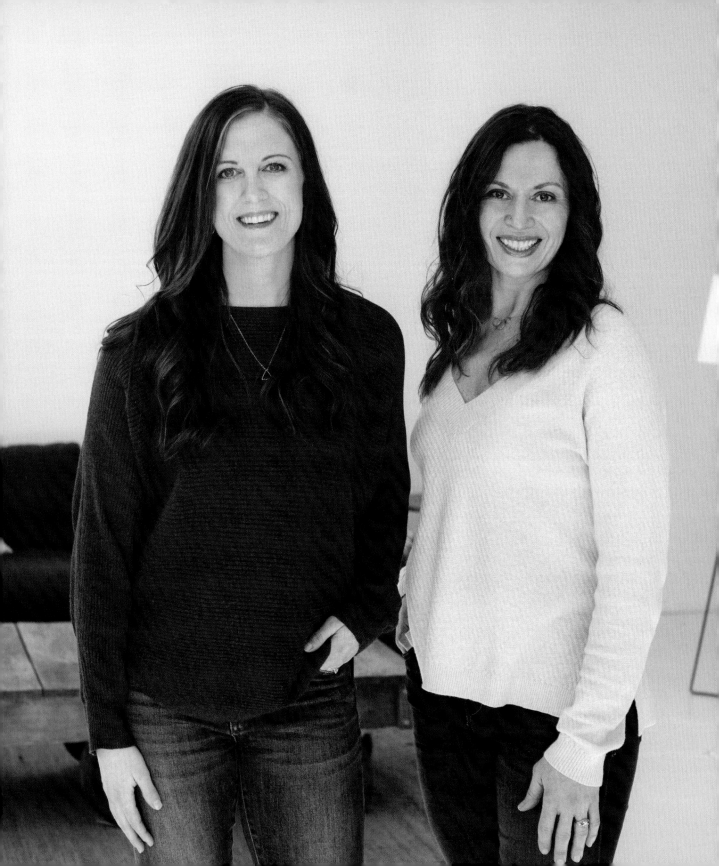

introduction

We met in New York City in June 2014 at an online business conference that neither of us really wanted to attend. We were already registered dietitians at the time—Jessica in Colorado and Stacie in Minnesota. What began as a plan to stay in touch with weekly phone calls and emails to help hold each other accountable to our individual business goals turned into an online meal-planning membership program that we started together. We quickly realized that wasn't for us, but we ultimately turned that business into a website to share recipes with our private practice nutrition clients and clinic patients. Today the website is our full-time job, with millions visiting the site each month looking for healthier versions of comfort foods or delicious recipes that fit their dietary needs or preferences.

This book is the result of what started as our little passion project and our way of giving back to our community of readers, friends, and family who have gathered at our virtual table over the years. *The Real Food Table* is a collection of recipes developed by us, focusing on whole and minimally processed foods. We believe that food is about more than calories and nutrients; it's about connection and creating lasting memories that nourish you long after the dishes are cleared.

We know you want to eat well and without a

lot of fuss. We hope that this collection of recipes will become family favorites and weeknight staples that you come back to again and again. Whether it's a busy weeknight, a relaxed weekend, or a holiday gathering that has you wondering what to cook, we've got a deliciously healthy, veggie-filled recipe for that.

our food philosophy

Everyone is welcome at our table. We believe that food is the ingredient that binds us together, so we seek to create meals that everyone can enjoy—no matter your budget, your dietary restrictions, or your taste buds. Throughout this book, you will find recipes that fit (or can be modified to fit) several different styles of eating, whether that be gluten-free, grain-free, dairy-free, nut-free, egg-free, or vegan. Buying organic is never a requirement, but if it's in your budget and important to you, then please, by all means choose organic ingredients. Organic agriculture is good for the health of humans, animals, and the environment, but if cost is an issue, do your best, keeping in mind that conventional produce is better than no produce at all when it comes to healthy eating. Additionally, we know that not everyone has easy access to specialty stores and foods—like Stacie, who lives in a rural location. For that reason, we've created these recipes using common ingredients that you can find any-place, whether you live in the heart of the city or the "middle of anywhere."

When it comes to diet and nutrition, our approach is anything but dogmatic. In fact, we believe that no one diet fits all and that all foods can fit into a healthy lifestyle. We both understand the challenges of balancing work and family life, and the difficulties that come with putting a nutritious meal on the table on busy weeknights. That's why the recipes in this book are not only healthy and delicious but simple to prepare. We give you shortcuts whenever possible, and if we can save you from washing extra bowls or pans, then we definitely will, because we know you have better things to do than spend the evening cleaning up.

While we do include nutrition information for every recipe, we don't promote calorie counting or restriction but rather using food for nourishment and enjoyment. Our goal has always been to help others eat mindfully and simply enjoy the food that they eat; to nourish their bodies in a sustainable way that makes them feel their best and ultimately enjoy life to the absolute fullest.

The following icons, found at the top of each recipe, will help you quickly identify whether or not a recipe fits your particular dietary style or needs or can be adapted to do so.

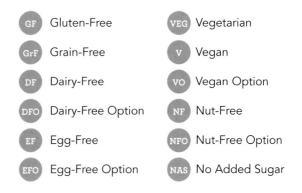

GF — Gluten-Free
GrF — Grain-Free
DF — Dairy-Free
DFO — Dairy-Free Option
EF — Egg-Free
EFO — Egg-Free Option
VEG — Vegetarian
V — Vegan
VO — Vegan Option
NF — Nut-Free
NFO — Nut-Free Option
NAS — No Added Sugar

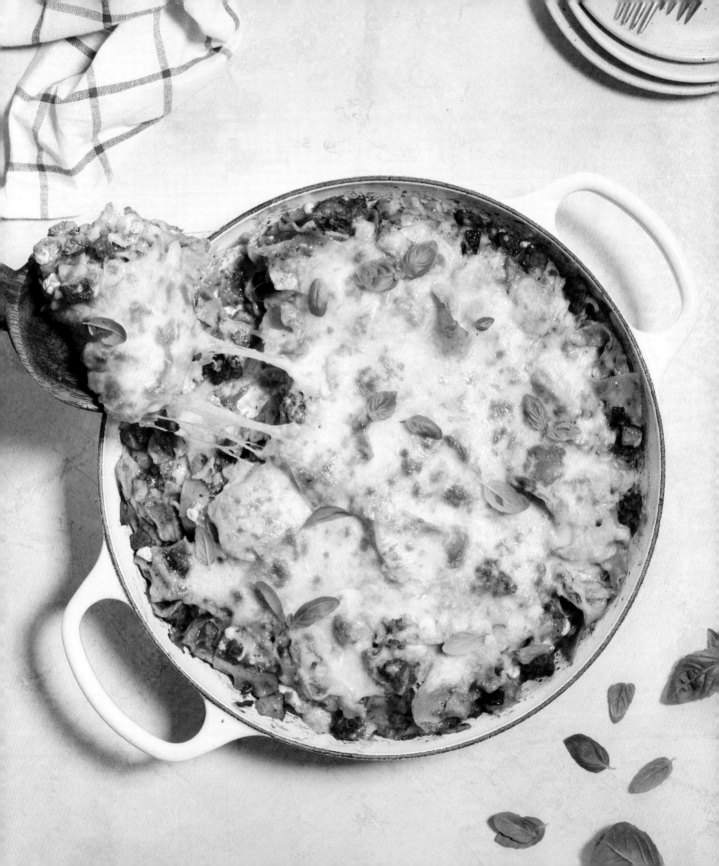

pantry staples

You'll notice ingredients we frequently use in our recipes throughout this book. These are the workhorse items that we like to have in our kitchens at all times. Having them on hand will make it easier to cook your way through the book and enjoy all that's to come in the pages ahead.

BEANS (CANNED): In all our recipes that call for canned beans, we use ones with no added salt. We always drain and rinse them beforehand to remove the starchy liquid.

BLACK PEPPER: Where we call for black pepper in the recipes, we are referring to ground black pepper in a bottle or a can. Freshly ground black pepper can also be used, but since it's more time-consuming to grind your own, we often save this kind for finishing dishes.

BROTH: We use low-sodium broth (whether it's chicken, beef, or vegetable) for all of our recipes because it allows us to add salt to taste and control the sodium level, which can get pretty high when using boxed broth.

COCONUT AMINOS: This gluten-free and soy-free alternative to soy sauce is made by blending the sap of coconut trees with sea salt, but it does not

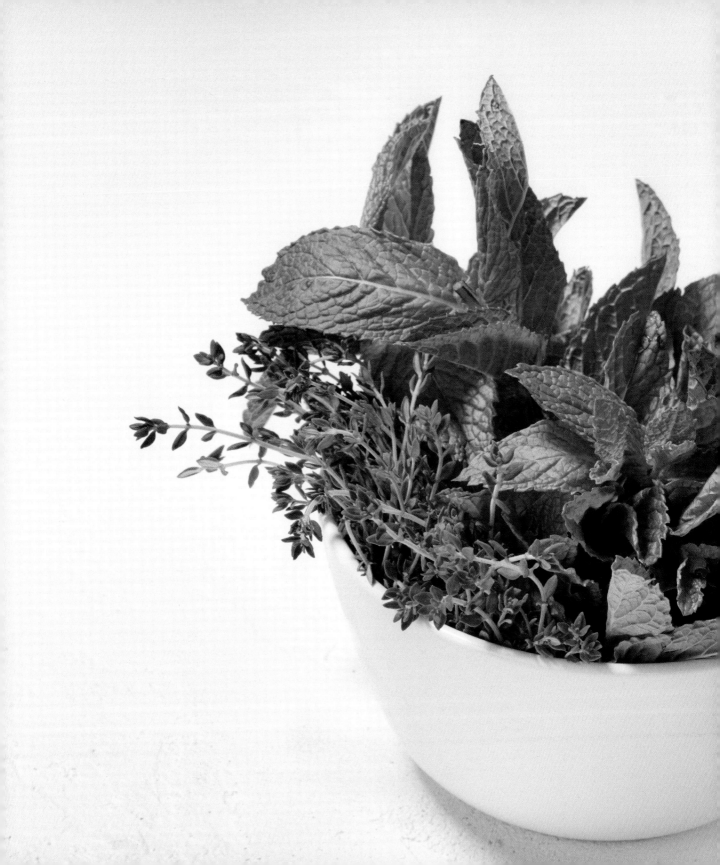

taste like coconut. Lower in sodium than most soy sauces, coconut aminos lend dishes a bit of natural sweetness without added sugar, which is why you'll see it used in recipes throughout the book.

COCONUT MILK (FULL-FAT): This is a creamy and delicious dairy-free alternative to milk and cream. While you might think that coconut milk will taste overwhelmingly like coconuts, the flavor is surprisingly subtle when added to savory soups and sauces, like our chicken corn chowder (page 77) and the mushroom-onion sauce for our smothered pork chops (page 152).

CORNSTARCH: A few of our sauce and stew recipes use cornstarch as a thickener. For a grain-free option, we specify the amount of arrowroot to use as a substitute.

GLUTEN-FREE ALL-PURPOSE FLOUR: Our go-to for baking is a gluten-free flour blend that can be used in a one-to-one ratio in place of wheat flour. Bob's Red Mill Gluten-Free 1-to-1 Baking Flour and King Arthur Gluten-Free All-Purpose Flour are two of our favorites.

MAYONNAISE: Use the best-quality mayonnaise, with the fewest ingredients, you can source. If you want to avoid added sugars, be sure to read the labels. Recipes calling for mayonnaise can be made egg-free by substituting vegan mayonnaise.

MUSTARD: Dijon and spicy brown mustard are great for adding flavor to sauces and dressings.

NONSTICK COOKING SPRAY: This spray in a can is a quick and easy way to keep foods from sticking to your pans. We also spritz it on crumb coatings before they go into the oven to make them a little extra crispy without having to fry in oil; see our Crispy Baked Chicken Nuggets (page 85) and Sheet Pan Fish-and-Chips (page 167).

NUT AND SEED BUTTERS: Peanut, almond, and cashew are our favorite nut butters. Many of the recipes in this book that call for nut butter can be made nut-free by substituting sunflower seed butter. We recommend using natural creamy nut butters (made with only nuts and salt) that have a slightly runny or drizzly consistency at room temperature. But if your nut butter has a thicker consistency, don't worry, we give tips in the recipes for how to use those, too.

OATS: If you need these recipes to be strictly gluten-free, be sure to use certified gluten-free oats. Check the package label for the certified gluten-free label, as not all oats are gluten-free due to processing on shared equipment and cross-contamination.

OILS: Avocado oil and extra-virgin olive oil are our go-tos and can be used interchangeably in almost any recipe. We like to cook with these oils because they're rich in heart-healthy fats. While we don't call for coconut oil in this book, we do offer it as a dairy-free alternative to butter in some of our recipes for baked and no-bake treats.

SALT: We use fine salt for cooking and baking in our recipes, and coarse sea salt and flaky sea salt, such as Maldon, for finishing.

SPICES: We keep our spice rack simple with a handful of regulars, and have found that with the right amount and combination of high-quality spices you don't need to have an extensive spice collection to create flavorful meals inspired by a variety of cuisines. The ones we turn to the most are garlic powder, onion powder, chili powder, ground cumin, smoked paprika, dried Italian seasoning, crushed red pepper flakes, dried thyme, and dried dill.

SWEETENERS: Yes, we sometimes call for brown sugar and granulated sugar in our recipes. But other times, we use honey or pure maple syrup to sweeten baked goods and add that little extra something to sauces, dressings, and marinades. The key is to use just enough sweetener to enhance and balance the other flavors, and add moisture to baked goods, while keeping the total amount of added sugar within reason.

TOMATO PASTE: Great for thickening or intensifying the flavor of other tomatoes in a soup, stew, or chili, tomato paste can also add a bit of savory richness to a marinade or sauce. You may find that you have leftover tomato paste when making our recipes, so freeze any leftover paste in one-tablespoon portions to use in future recipes, or purchase it in a tube so you can squeeze out just what you need and store the rest in the refrigerator.

TOMATOES (CANNED): We always keep a variety of canned tomato products like whole peeled, diced, crushed, fire-roasted diced, and tomato sauce in our pantries because they're so versatile and easier to use than fresh tomatoes when making sauces, soups, and stews. Plus, canned tomatoes are always in season. We don't specify "no added salt" for these ingredients, but feel free to use them and adjust the salt in the recipe to suit your taste.

VINEGAR: Vinegar has so many uses in cooking, from adding a lovely tang to dressings and sauces to balancing flavors in savory dishes to giving a lift to baked goods. It's an ingredient that should be in every pantry. We most commonly use apple cider vinegar, rice vinegar, balsamic, and red wine vinegar.

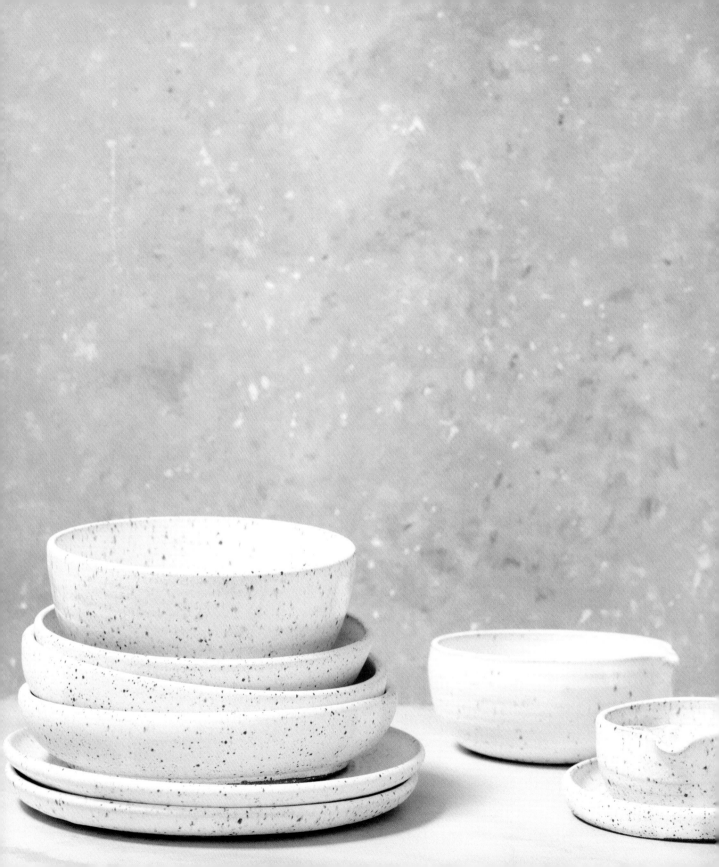

kitchen essentials

When it comes to kitchen essentials, we like to keep things to a minimum. This list includes our go-to tools and equipment—the ones we use most frequently in the recipes throughout this book. Most of the items you'll likely already have on hand. While not all of these tools and equipment are required to make the recipes, they will definitely help get the job done more efficiently, which is why we recommend them for every kitchen.

BAKING DISH (9×9-INCH AND 9×13-INCH): When we call for a baking dish in recipes like the One-Bowl Mixed Berry Crisp (page 229), Apple Cobbler (page 234), and Sloppy Joe Casserole (page 146), we are referring to a glass or ceramic dish.

BAKING PAN (8×8-INCH): When we call for a baking pan in recipes like our Peanut Butter Swirl Brownies (page 241), Jammy Blueberry Pie Bars (page 231), and One-Bowl Chocolate Chip Blondies (page 243), we are referring to a metal baking pan. You could substitute a glass or ceramic baking dish, but it will increase the baking time slightly, depending on the recipe.

BAKING SHEETS: Rimmed baking sheets can be used for anything from making cookies to sheet pan meals to protecting your oven floor from spill-overs. We have found that one is never enough, three might be too many, but two is just right. We recommend the 11×17-inch size.

BLENDER (HIGH-POWERED): A high-powered blender, though an investment, is an invaluable tool for whipping up smoothies, blending soups, and making creamy dairy-free sauces from nuts. We like the Vitamix brand because it's easy to use, extremely powerful, and well made so it will last for many years.

FOOD PROCESSOR: Don't underestimate the value of a food processor. Not only is it a timesaver for chopping and mincing, it makes quick work of crushing tortilla chips into crumbs to coat chicken or fish. When fitted with a slicing or shredding blade, a food processor can cut down signifi-cantly on prep time for salads and slaws.

INSTANT POT: Getting dinner on the table fast when you didn't plan ahead is where the Instant Pot really shines. This is one of our favorite appli-ances because it has so many uses, from making a big batch of Busy Morning Oatmeal Two Ways (page 24) to Instant Pot Garlic Mashed Potatoes (page 62) to tender Instant Pot Pulled Pork (page 155) that you can pile into sandwiches.

KITCHEN SCALE (DIGITAL): A digital kitchen scale is super helpful for weighing ingredients like meat, cheese, and vegetables that are otherwise difficult to measure accurately with measuring cups or spoons. It's also useful for weighing our recommended serving sizes of cooked proteins, like Slow Cooker Tacos al Pastor (page 129), In-stant Pot Beef Barbacoa Burrito Bowls (page 123), and Instant Pot Pulled Pork (page 155).

KITCHEN SHEARS: This handy kitchen tool is extremely useful for trimming meats, snipping herbs, opening packages, and more.

KNIVES: A set of high-quality knives will make cooking much more enjoyable. These are our must-have and most-used knives for everyday cooking: a chef's (or cook's) knife for cutting large pieces of meat and dicing or slicing vegetables; a bread or serrated knife for slicing soft vegetables like tomatoes and, of course, bread; a utility knife (a larger version of a paring knife) for times when a chef's knife is too big for the job, like deboning whole chicken or trimming fat from meat; and a paring knife for more precise tasks, like halving cherry tomatoes, berries, and grapes, or remov-ing the core from a sliced apple.

MICROPLANE: We have found this do-it-all gad-get indispensable in the kitchen for zesting citrus fruits, as well as grating hard cheeses, chocolate, garlic, and ginger.

PARCHMENT PAPER: Do you like easy cleanup? Then get yourself a roll of parchment paper. Lin-ing baking sheets for sheet pan meals saves you from scrubbing burned-on messes. Parchment paper is also essential for lining baking pans to keep cakes from sticking, and easily lifting brown-ies and bars from the pan.

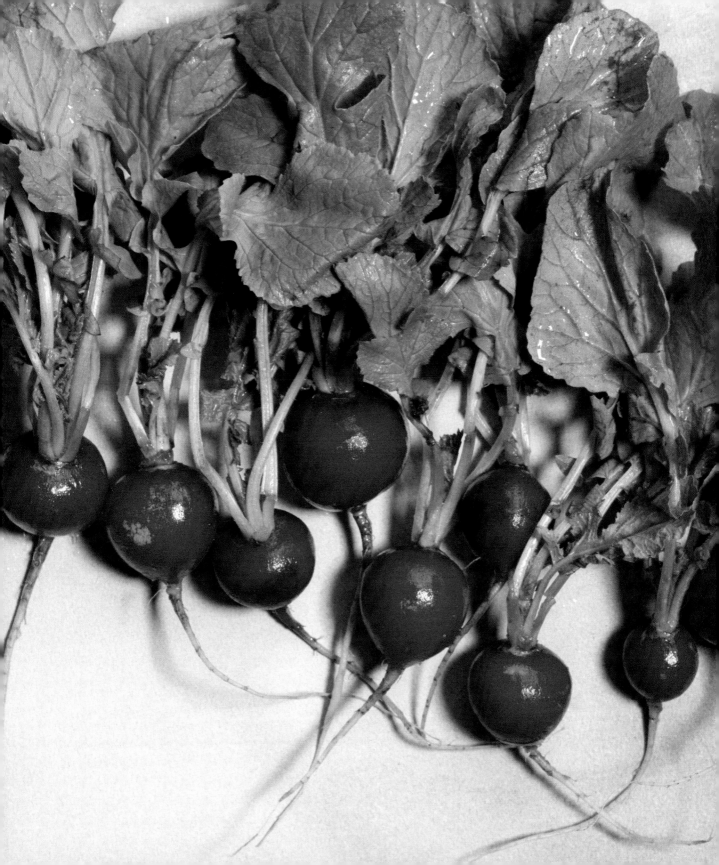

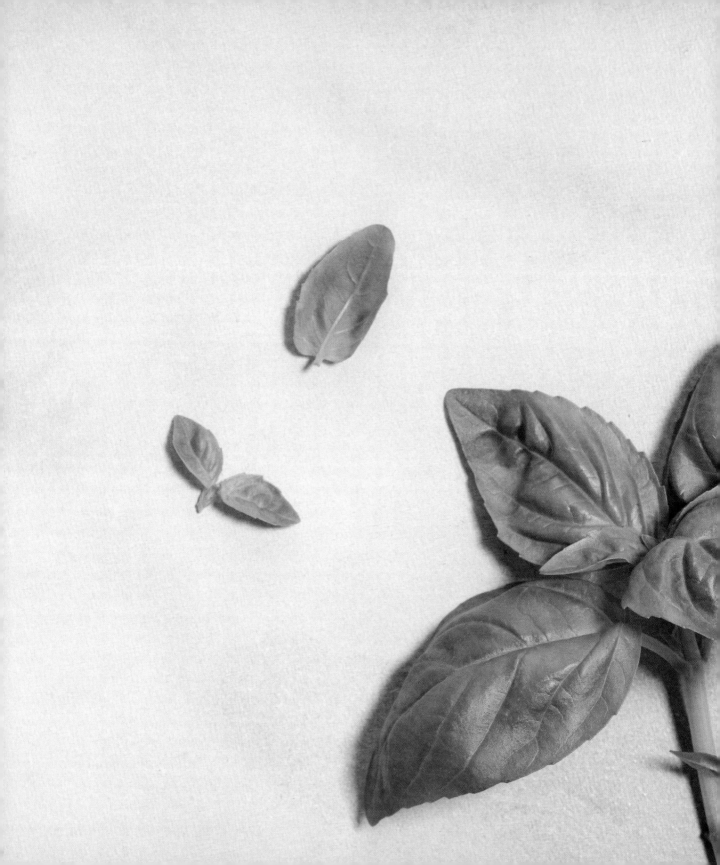

POTS, PANS, AND SKILLETS: We would consider these to be the essentials for any kitchen:

- A 5- to 6-quart round or oval Dutch oven is vital for making soups and stews, and slow-cooking meat in the oven when a slow cooker is not available.
- 2- and 3-quart saucepans with lids (which we refer to as "medium" in our recipes) are what we use to cook smaller amounts of vegetables and sauces, and for boiling eggs.
- A 12-inch cast-iron skillet with a lid or a 3½-quart enameled cast-iron casserole dish with a lid (also known as a "braiser"; Lodge makes a very affordable one). This is our go-to vessel for stir-fries, breakfast hashes, one-skillet meals, and more. It's also great for browning meat before adding it to the slow cooker to give the meat extra flavor.

SLOW COOKER: Slow cookers are where it's at when you want a meal with minimal fuss. With just a little prep, you can fill the slow cooker with ingredients in the morning and come home to a meal that's hot and ready when you walk in the door, like our Slow Cooker White Chicken Chili with White Beans (page 75), Slow Cooker Irish Beef Stew (page 119), and Slow Cooker Tacos al Pastor (page 129).

STAND MIXER OR HAND MIXER: While not absolutely necessary, it sure makes creaming butter and sugar a whole lot easier when making cookies and bars. Either appliance will save you from whisking forever by hand when whipping cream.

THERMOMETER (INSTANT-READ DIGITAL): Is the meat overcooked or underdone? The only way to really know is by using a thermometer to check the internal temperature of the meat you're cooking. Stop guessing and get an instant-read thermometer, which registers a quick digital temperature. It's inexpensive, easy to use, and you'll be a better cook for it.

THERMOMETER (OVEN): If you set your oven temperature to 350°F, that's the temperature it will be inside, right? Not necessarily. It's not uncommon for ovens to vary in temperature by 5°F to 25°F, so having a thermometer in the oven that gives you an accurate reading can help you achieve the correct temperature for the best results when baking and roasting.

VEGETABLE PEELER: These are best for removing skins on fruits and vegetables or to easily shave vegetables into ribbons, like we do for our Quick-Pickled Carrots or Cucumbers (page 267).

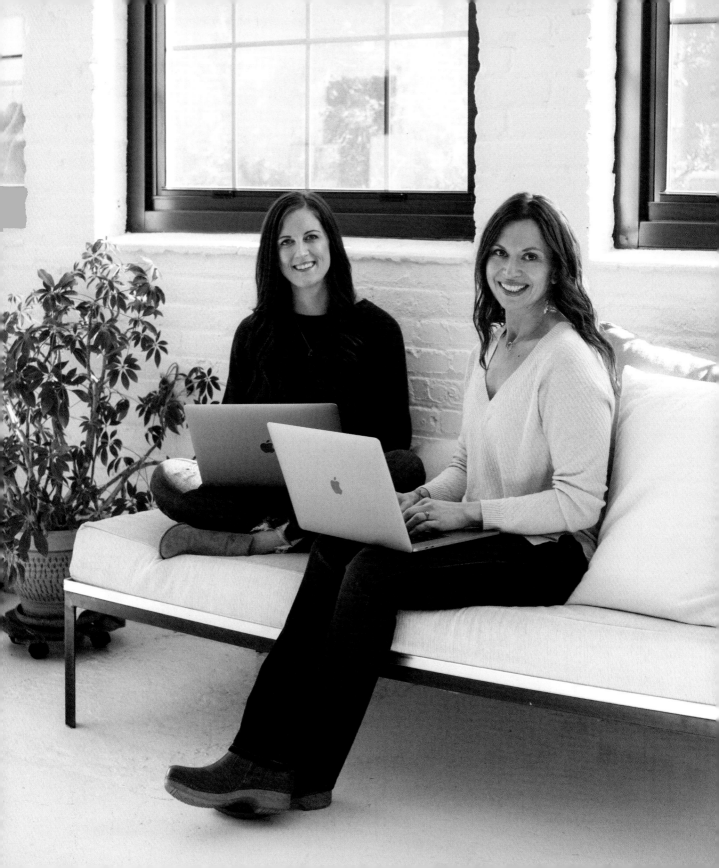

four-week dinner plan

What's for dinner? To help you answer this daunting question, we created a four-week dinner plan based on recipes from this book. Our goal was to make a realistic plan for you so you don't have to find a new recipe for every night of the week. We focused on what tends to be the biggest impediment when it comes to meal planning: dinners. We chose four recipes to make each week. You can then fill the gaps with leftovers or "clean out the refrigerator" meals or takeout. We promise, you'll look forward to the leftovers.

Make this meal plan work for you! Feel free to move the recipes around to fit your schedule, and if there's a dish in the book you're especially excited about, go ahead and swap it in.

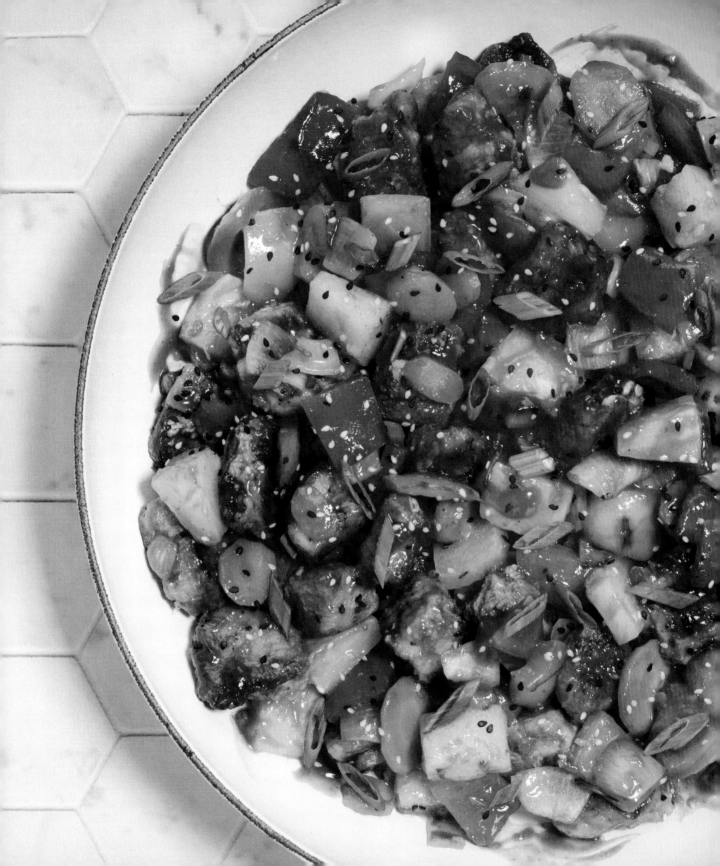

Week 1

MEAL 1	MEAL 2	MEAL 3	MEAL 4
Slow Cooker White Chicken Chili with White Beans (page 75)	Sheet Pan Mini Meat Loaf Dinner (page 139)	Slow Cooker Tacos al Pastor (page 129)	Egg Bake with Sweet Potatoes & Turkey Sausage (page 30)

Week 2

MEAL 1	MEAL 2	MEAL 3	MEAL 4
Sheet Pan Honey-Garlic Chicken & Vegetables with Goat Cheese Sauce (page 89)	Beef & Broccoli (& Then Some!) (page 131)	Fish Tacos with Avocado "Crema" (page 169)	Rainbow Quinoa Bowls with Peanut Dressing (page 183)

Week 3

MEAL 1	MEAL 2	MEAL 3	MEAL 4
Slow Cooker or Instant Pot Chicken Corn Chowder (page 77)	Sheet Pan Steak Fajitas (page 127)	Sweet-&-Sour Pork (page 151)	Chicken Sausage & Sweet Potato Skillet Hash (page 33)

Week 4

MEAL 1	MEAL 2	MEAL 3	MEAL 4
Easy Egg Roll Bowls (page 107)	Shredded Barbecue Beef–Stuffed Sweet Potatoes (page 135)	Sheet Pan Harissa Salmon with Vegetables (page 171)	Minestrone Soup (page 180)

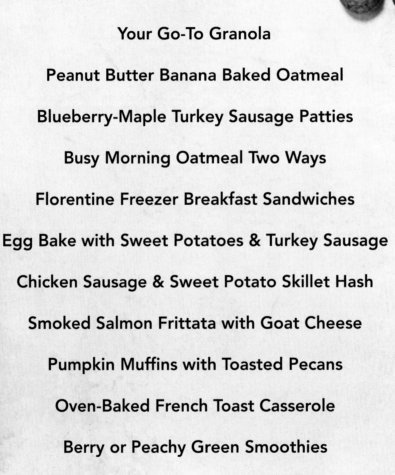

Your Go-To Granola

Peanut Butter Banana Baked Oatmeal

Blueberry-Maple Turkey Sausage Patties

Busy Morning Oatmeal Two Ways

Florentine Freezer Breakfast Sandwiches

Egg Bake with Sweet Potatoes & Turkey Sausage

Chicken Sausage & Sweet Potato Skillet Hash

Smoked Salmon Frittata with Goat Cheese

Pumpkin Muffins with Toasted Pecans

Oven-Baked French Toast Casserole

Berry or Peachy Green Smoothies

breakfast
& brunch

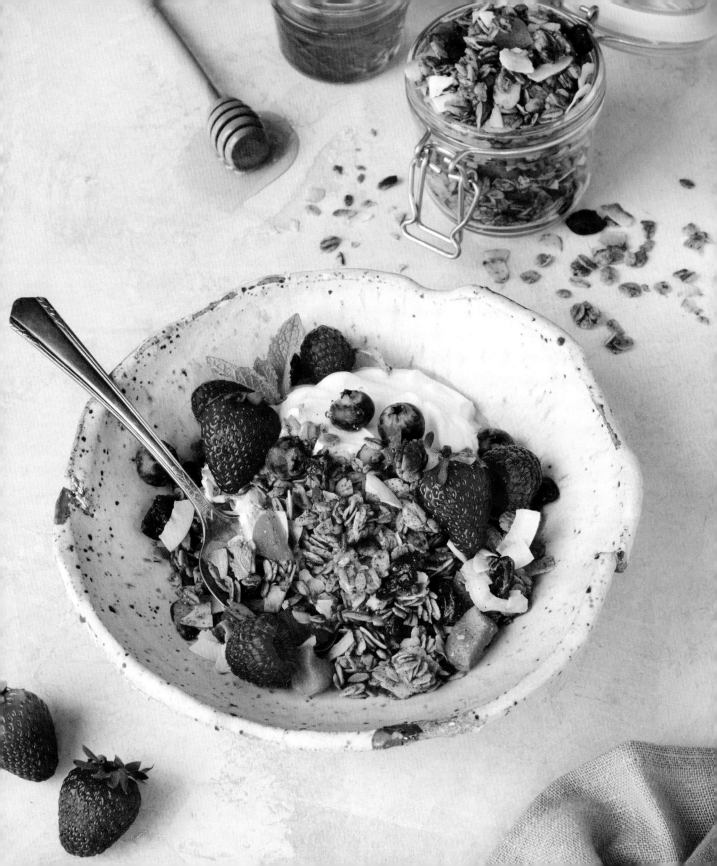

your go-to granola

Prep Time: **15 minutes** | Cook Time: **25 minutes** | Total Time: **40 minutes** | Makes **5 cups (15 servings)**

GF
DF
EF
V

2½ cups old-fashioned rolled oats
½ cup unsweetened coconut flakes
½ cup sliced raw almonds
¼ cup avocado oil or melted coconut oil
½ cup pure maple syrup
2 teaspoons ground cinnamon
2 teaspoons pure vanilla extract
⅛ teaspoon fine salt
¾ cup dried fruit of choice, such as raisins, cranberries, cherries, chopped figs, apricots, or dates

We love granola, but we don't always love the ingredients or the price tag on those little bags at the store. Making your own granola is easy, allows you to control what goes into it, and is budget friendly. This granola is great added to yogurt, swirled into a smoothie, or served with your favorite milk and fresh fruit. Feel free to customize your granola using whatever nuts and dried fruit you have on hand.

Preheat the oven to 300°F. Line a rimmed baking sheet with parchment paper or a silicone baking mat and set aside.

In a medium bowl, combine the oats, coconut flakes, and almonds. In a separate small bowl, whisk the avocado oil, maple syrup, cinnamon, vanilla, and salt. Pour over the oat mixture and stir to combine.

Spread the unbaked granola evenly on the prepared baking sheet and bake for 25 to 30 minutes, without stirring, or until the granola is lightly browned.

Remove from the oven and allow the granola to cool completely on the baking sheet, then break into clusters and gently combine with the dried fruit.

Serve, as desired, or store the granola in an airtight container at room temperature for up to 3 weeks.

Tips from the Dietitians
Homemade granola makes a great gift when packaged in small bags or jars and tied with a ribbon.

Nutrition Info: (Serving size: ⅓ cup) 188 calories, 8g total fat, 2g saturated fat, 22mg sodium, 27g carbs, 12g sugar, 3g fiber, 4g protein

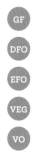

GF

DFO

EFO

VEG

VO

peanut butter banana baked oatmeal

Prep Time: **10 minutes** | Cook Time: **35 minutes** | Total Time: **45 minutes** | Makes **9 servings**

Nonstick cooking spray
2½ cups old-fashioned rolled oats
1 teaspoon ground cinnamon
½ teaspoon baking powder
¼ teaspoon fine salt
2 overripe bananas, mashed
½ cup natural creamy peanut
    butter
1 large egg (use a flax egg, for
    vegan and egg-free; see Tips)
2 tablespoons pure maple syrup
1 teaspoon pure vanilla extract
1 cup milk (or nondairy milk, for
    dairy-free and vegan)

Optional toppings:
Banana slices or other fresh fruit,
    peanut butter, pure maple
    syrup, yogurt, and/or milk or
    nondairy milk

Baked oatmeal is super easy to make. One advantage of baking oatmeal is that you make it ahead to enjoy for breakfast or a snack throughout the week (served warm or cold). It's also a great addition to lunch boxes. The texture is similar to a very soft breakfast bar. Try it topped with yogurt, peanut butter, fresh fruit, and/or a drizzle of maple syrup or honey for something extra delicious. You can also serve the baked oatmeal in a bowl with a little milk poured over the top.

Preheat the oven to 350°F. Spray a 9×9-inch baking dish with cooking spray and set aside.

In a medium bowl, combine the oats, cinnamon, baking powder, and salt. Add the mashed banana, peanut butter, egg, maple syrup, and vanilla and stir. Then add the milk and stir until well combined. Transfer to the prepared baking dish and spread out into an even layer.

Bake for 30 to 35 minutes, or until the center of the oatmeal is set and lightly firm to the touch. Allow to cool for 10 minutes before serving.

Serve with your desired toppings.

Store leftovers in an airtight container or large zip-top bag in the refrigerator for up to 1 week or freeze up to 3 months.

> Tips from the Dietitians
>
> To make a flax egg, stir 1 tablespoon of ground flaxseed into
> 3 tablespoons of water in a small bowl until well combined and let
> stand for 5 minutes. Use it in place of the 1 large egg in the recipe.
>
> For a little something sweet, mix in a handful of chocolate chips after
> stirring in the milk.

Nutrition Info: (Serving size: ⅑ of the recipe without the optional toppings) 237 calories, 10g total fat, 2g saturated fat, 142mg sodium, 30g carbs, 7g sugar, 4g fiber, 9g protein

blueberry-maple turkey sausage patties

Prep Time: **15 minutes** | Cook Time: **15 minutes** | Total Time: **30 minutes** | Makes **4 servings**

GF
GrF
DF
EF
NF

1 pound lean ground turkey (we use 93% lean/7% fat)
1 tablespoon pure maple syrup
¾ teaspoon ground sage
¾ teaspoon fine salt
½ teaspoon garlic powder
¼ teaspoon ground cinnamon
¼ teaspoon ground black pepper
½ cup fresh blueberries
1 tablespoon avocado oil or extra-virgin olive oil, divided

If you've never made your own breakfast sausage, now is the time to give it a try. These patties are easy to make, free of preservatives and additives, and the blueberries and cinnamon combined with sage make them both sweet and savory. They're the perfect pairing for eggs, oatmeal, a smoothie, or a stack of fluffy pancakes.

In a medium bowl, combine the turkey, maple syrup, sage, salt, garlic powder, cinnamon, and pepper. Mix thoroughly, being careful not to overmix. Gently fold in the blueberries.

Using a spoon or cookie scoop, scoop the mixture into 12 (1½-ounce) portions. With wet hands, form the mixture into patties about ¼ inch thick and 2 inches in diameter.

Place a large skillet over medium heat. When hot, add ½ tablespoon of the avocado oil and swirl to coat the bottom. Add half of the patties, being careful not to crowd them. Cook until browned and cooked through, 3 to 4 minutes per side. Transfer the patties to a plate and repeat with the remaining ½ tablespoon oil and patties.

Serve the sausage patties right away or store in an airtight container in the refrigerator for up to 4 days or freeze for up to 1 month.

Tips from the Dietitians
Shaping the sausage mixture into small patties makes them easier to flip when cooking and helps them stay together so you don't lose any of those juicy blueberries to the pan.

Nutrition Info: (Serving size: 3 patties) 194 calories, 9g total fat, 2g saturated fat, 523mg sodium, 6g carbs, 5g sugar, 1g fiber, 20g protein

busy morning oatmeal two ways

Prep Time: **5 minutes** | Cook Time: **varies** | Total Time **(Instant Pot): 40 minutes, includes 30 minutes for pressure buildup and natural release** | Total Time **(slow cooker): 4 hours 5 minutes** | Makes **6 servings**

1½ cup steel-cut oats

3 cups milk (or nondairy milk, for dairy-free and vegan)

2 cups water, if using an Instant Pot (or 3 cups water, if using a slow cooker)

⅛ teaspoon fine salt

2 teaspoons pure vanilla extract

Optional toppings:

In-season fruits or thawed frozen fruit, honey (omit for vegan) or pure maple syrup, ground cinnamon, chopped nuts and/or nut butter (omit for nut-free)

We call this Busy Morning Oatmeal because it only requires five minutes of hands-on time, leaving you free to take care of your morning routine, walk the dog, or find that missing shoe for the third time this week. You can prepare this oatmeal in an Instant Pot or a slow cooker, so no matter what your morning looks like, you've got an option.

Instant Pot Directions

In a 6-quart Instant Pot, combine the oats, milk, water, and salt and stir to mix. Lock the lid in place and switch the valve to the "sealing" position. Set the Instant Pot to cook at high pressure for 6 minutes. It will take about 10 minutes for the Instant Pot to build up the pressure before the timer starts counting down.

When the timer goes off, allow the pressure to naturally release for 15 minutes. Switch the valve to "venting" after the natural release time is up. Once the venting time is complete, remove the lid and stir in the vanilla.

Serve the oatmeal with your desired toppings. Store leftovers in an airtight container in the refrigerator for up to 5 days.

Slow Cooker Directions

Place the oats, milk, water, and salt in a 4- to 6-quart slow cooker and stir to mix. Cover and cook on low for 4 hours.

Uncover and stir in the vanilla.

Serve the oatmeal with your desired toppings. Store leftovers in an airtight container in the refrigerator for up to 5 days.

Nutrition Info: (Serving size: about 1 cup without the optional toppings) 232 calories, 4g total fat, 2g saturated fat, 108mg sodium, 37g carbs, 7g sugar, 4g fiber, 10g protein

Tips from the Dietitians

The oatmeal can be made ahead on the weekend for an easy reheat-and-eat breakfast option during the week.

To reheat in the microwave: Place the oatmeal in a microwave-safe bowl and microwave for 60 seconds. Stir and microwave for an additional 30 to 60 seconds at a time until the oatmeal is heated through.

To reheat on the stovetop: Place the oatmeal in a small saucepan with a splash of your milk of choice or water. Cook over medium-low heat, stirring occasionally, until heated through, 3 to 5 minutes.

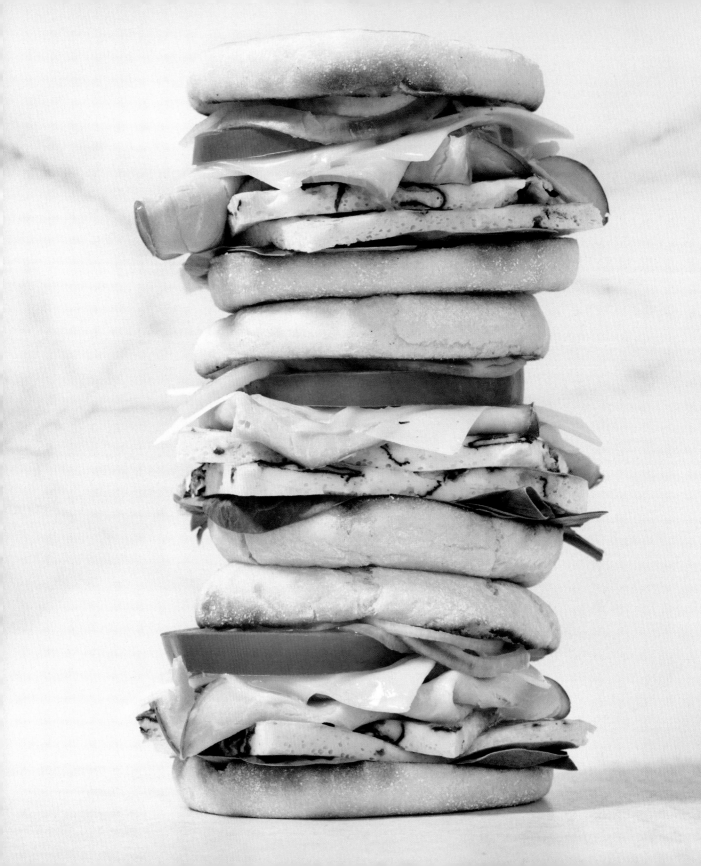

florentine freezer breakfast sandwiches

Prep Time: **30 minutes** | Cook Time: **25 minutes** | Total Time: **55 minutes, plus 5 minutes for cooling** | Makes **12 servings**

GFO
DFO
NF
NAS

Butter (or nonstick cooking spray, for dairy-free), for greasing
1 teaspoon avocado oil or extra-virgin olive oil
½ medium yellow onion, finely diced (1 cup)
18 large eggs
⅓ cup milk (or nondairy milk, for dairy-free)
¼ teaspoon fine salt
⅛ teaspoon ground black pepper
1 garlic clove, minced
5 cups loosely packed baby spinach (5 ounces)
12 gluten-free English muffins or bagels, split and toasted
4 ounces sliced deli ham (12 slices)
12 slices Swiss cheese (omit for dairy-free)

Optional toppings:
Sliced tomatoes, fresh baby spinach, red onion, sliced or mashed avocado, and/or hot sauce

If you've ever wanted a warm breakfast sandwich to take on your morning commute or on your next big adventure, then this recipe is for you! The best part (other than the spinach-studded egg patty, Swiss cheese, and savory ham sandwiched between a soft English muffin) is that you can make a big batch ahead and stash them in the freezer, then reheat them as needed. Jessica keeps her freezer stocked with these so they're ready to grab, reheat, and go for early morning adventures in the mountains.

Preheat the oven to 350°F. Grease an 11x17-inch rimmed baking sheet generously with butter and set aside.

Place a large skillet over medium heat. When hot, add the avocado oil and swirl to coat the bottom. Add the onion and cook, stirring occasionally, until it softens, 7 to 8 minutes.

Meanwhile, whisk the eggs and milk in a large bowl. Season with the salt and pepper, and set aside.

Stir the garlic into the onion and cook for another minute. Add the spinach and cook, stirring or tossing, until the spinach starts to wilt, 1 to 2 minutes.

Pour the eggs into the prepared baking sheet, then top with the spinach and onion mixture, spreading it out evenly.

Bake for 10 to 12 minutes, or until the egg is set and slightly puffed and no longer jiggly in the center. Remove the baking sheet from the oven and allow the eggs to cool for 5 to 10 minutes.

While the eggs are baking, place the English muffin bottoms, split side up, on another baking sheet or a cutting board. Top each with 1 slice of the ham and 1 slice of the cheese.

Continued on the next page

When the eggs have cooled slightly, use a knife to cut them into 24 equal portions. Add 2 egg portions to each sandwich, then close with the English muffin tops.

Serve right away, or if freezing for later, allow the egg sandwiches to cool for 20 minutes, then wrap each one tightly with aluminum foil. Transfer the wrapped sandwiches to a large zip-top bag or an airtight container and store in the freezer for up to 3 months.

Tips from the Dietitians

To reheat the sandwiches from thawed: Place the desired number of sandwiches in the refrigerator to thaw overnight, then bake, wrapped, in a preheated 350°F oven or toaster oven for about 20 minutes, or until heated through. To reheat in the microwave, remove and discard the foil. Wrap loosely in a paper towel and microwave for 1½ to 2 minutes, or until heated through.

To reheat the sandwiches from frozen: Bake the wrapped breakfast sandwich(es) in a preheated 350°F oven or toaster oven for 30 to 35 minutes, or until heated through. To reheat in the microwave, remove and discard the foil. Wrap loosely in a paper towel and microwave for 3 minutes, or until heated through.

Feel free to change up the fillings with different vegetables, breakfast meat, or cheese to make these sandwiches your own.

Nutrition Info: (Serving size: 1 sandwich without the optional toppings) 314 calories, 13g total fat, 6g saturated fat, 514mg sodium, 29g carbs, 6g sugar, 2g fiber, 21g protein

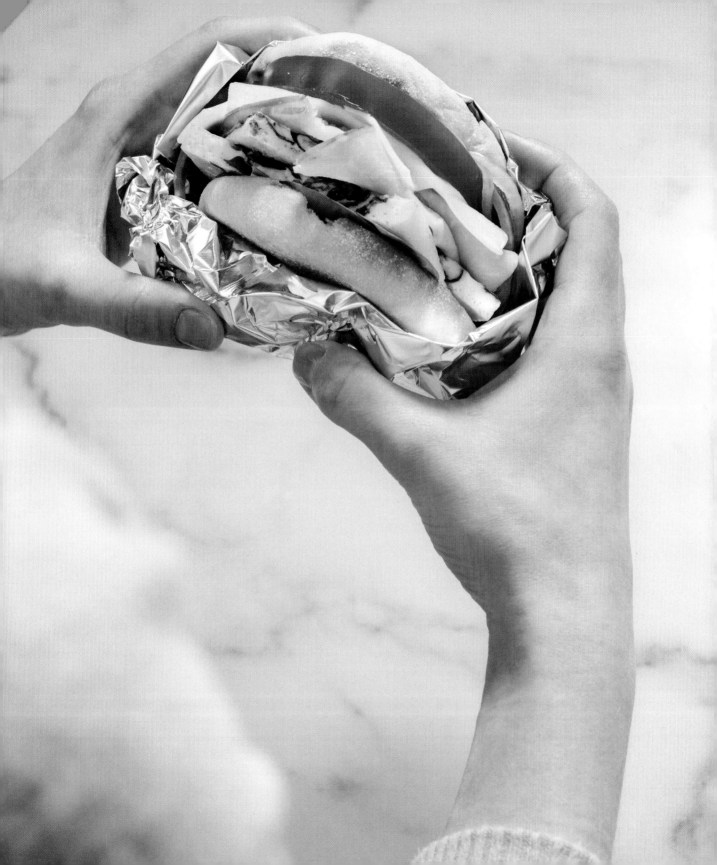

egg bake with sweet potatoes & turkey sausage

Prep Time: **20 minutes** | Cook Time: **20 minutes** | Total Time: **40 minutes, plus 5 minutes standing time** | Makes **8**

GF
GrF
DFO
NF
NAS

1 tablespoon plus 2 teaspoons avocado oil or extra-virgin olive oil, divided, plus more for greasing (or use nonstick cooking spray)

1 pound lean ground turkey (we use 93% lean/7% fat)

2 teaspoons dried Italian seasoning

1 teaspoon garlic powder

1 teaspoon fennel seeds, crushed (see Tips)

1½ teaspoons fine salt, plus more as needed

½ teaspoon ground black pepper, plus more as needed

2 medium to large sweet potatoes, peeled and cut into ¼-inch cubes (4 to 4½ cups)

½ medium red onion, diced (1 cup)

1 medium red bell pepper, diced (1 cup)

5 cups loosely packed baby spinach (5 ounces)

12 large eggs

½ cup milk (or nondairy milk, for dairy-free)

1 cup shredded cheese of choice (omit for dairy-free)

Optional toppings:
Sliced avocado and/or hot sauce

This hearty breakfast casserole uses sweet potatoes and a variety of vegetables in place of the usual bread to add a healthy dose of fiber and vitamins. The homemade sausage, which is easy to make, is just like the bulk sausage you buy at the grocery store, only it's free of preservatives, added sugars, colors, and flavors. This egg bake is a great way to use up the random bits of vegetables in your crisper, and when made ahead, it's a delicious reheat-and-eat option for any time of the day.

Preheat the oven to 375°F. Grease a 9×13-inch baking dish generously with avocado oil or cooking spray, and set aside.

To make the homemade turkey sausage, place a large skillet over medium-high heat. When hot, add the 2 teaspoons of oil and swirl to coat the bottom. Add the turkey, Italian seasoning, garlic powder, fennel seeds, 1 teaspoon of the salt, and ¼ teaspoon of the black pepper. Break up the turkey with a wooden spoon and cook, stirring occasionally, until browned and cooked through, 5 to 6 minutes. Transfer the turkey sausage to the prepared baking dish.

To the same skillet (no need to wipe it out first), add the 1 tablespoon oil and swirl to coat the bottom. Add the sweet potatoes and cook, stirring occasionally, for 10 minutes.

Add the onion and bell pepper to the sweet potatoes in the skillet. Add a dash each of salt and pepper and cook, stirring occasionally, until the sweet potatoes are tender, 5 to 6 minutes. Add the spinach with a splash of water (about 2 tablespoons) and cook, stirring occasionally, until the spinach is wilted, 2 to 3 minutes.

Transfer the vegetables to the baking dish, spreading them out over the turkey sausage.

In a medium bowl, whisk the eggs, milk, the remaining ½ teaspoon salt, and the remaining ¼ teaspoon black pepper. Stir in the cheese. Pour the eggs over the turkey sausage and vegetables. With the back of a wooden spoon, submerge the vegetables under the eggs as much as possible.

Bake for 18 to 22 minutes, or until the center of the egg bake is set. Remove from the oven and let stand for 5 minutes before serving.

Cut the egg bake into 8 pieces. Add salt and pepper to taste. Top with sliced avocado or a drizzle of hot sauce, if desired, and serve.

Store leftovers in an airtight container in the refrigerator for up to 4 days or in the freezer for up to 3 months.

Tips from the Dietitians
Cutting the sweet potato into small cubes decreases the cooking time.

To crush the fennel seeds, use a mortar and pestle. Alternatively, move the flat side of a large chef's knife blade over the fennel seeds, pressing down with your fingertips to crush the seeds lightly.

To reheat in the microwave: Place the egg bake on a microwave-safe plate and microwave for 90 seconds. Touch the center of the egg bake with your finger. If it's not hot, microwave for 30 seconds at a time until hot to touch.

To reheat on the stovetop: Add the egg bake and 1 to 2 tablespoons of water to a skillet over medium heat. Cover and cook until heated through, 4 to 5 minutes.

Nutrition Info: (Serving size: ⅛ of the recipe) 341 calories, 16g total fat, 6g saturated fat, 714mg sodium, 26g carbs, 4g sugar, 4g fiber, 24g protein

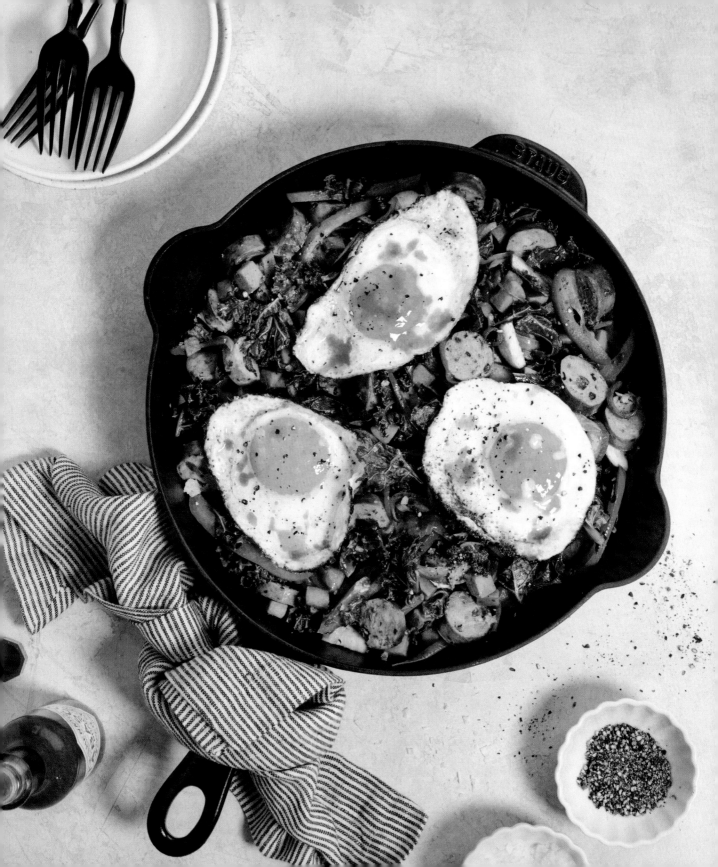

chicken sausage & sweet potato skillet hash

Prep Time: **20 minutes** | Cook Time: **25 minutes** | Total Time: **45 minutes** | Makes **4 servings**

GF · GrF · DF · EFO · NF · NAS

1 tablespoon avocado oil or extra-virgin olive oil

1 medium to large sweet potato, peeled and cut into ¼-inch cubes (2 to 2½ cups)

Fine salt and ground black pepper

1 medium red bell pepper, sliced (1 cup)

½ medium red onion, sliced (1 cup)

1 small zucchini, halved or quartered lengthwise then sliced crosswise ½ inch thick (1 cup)

4 cups chopped curly kale

12 to 14 ounces fully cooked chicken sausage links, sliced ½ inch thick

Optional toppings:
Fried egg (omit for egg-free), sliced avocado, and/or hot sauce

Made all in one skillet, this veggie- and protein-packed breakfast is guaranteed to satisfy even the heartiest of appetites, with or without a fried egg on top. Reheated leftovers taste great, making this a perfect weekend meal prep recipe. This is also a great way to use up the random vegetable bits and pieces hanging out in the crisper. Feel free to swap out the red bell pepper, onion, and/or zucchini with vegetables you have on hand.

Place a large skillet over medium-high heat. When hot, add the avocado oil and swirl to coat the bottom. Add the sweet potato and a pinch each of salt and pepper. Cook, stirring occasionally, for about 12 minutes.

Add the remaining vegetables, the sausage, and a pinch each of salt and pepper to the skillet. Cook, stirring occasionally, until the sweet potato is tender and cooked through, 12 to 14 minutes.

Serve the hash warm. Top with a fried egg, sliced avocado, and/or a drizzle of hot sauce, if desired. Add salt and pepper to taste.

Store leftovers in an airtight container in the refrigerator for up to 4 days.

Tips from the Dietitians

If prepping ahead, portion the hash in individual, microwave-safe glass containers for an easy grab-and-go meal that you can reheat.

To reheat in the microwave: Place the hash in a microwave-safe container and microwave for 60 seconds then stir. If it's not hot, continue to heat for 30 seconds at a time until hot to touch.

If you're looking to avoid added sugars, use chicken sausage made without sugar.

Nutrition Info: (Serving size: 1½ cups without additional toppings) 300 calories, 12g total fat, 3g saturated fat, 594mg sodium, 28g carbs, 14g sugar, 5g fiber, 21g protein

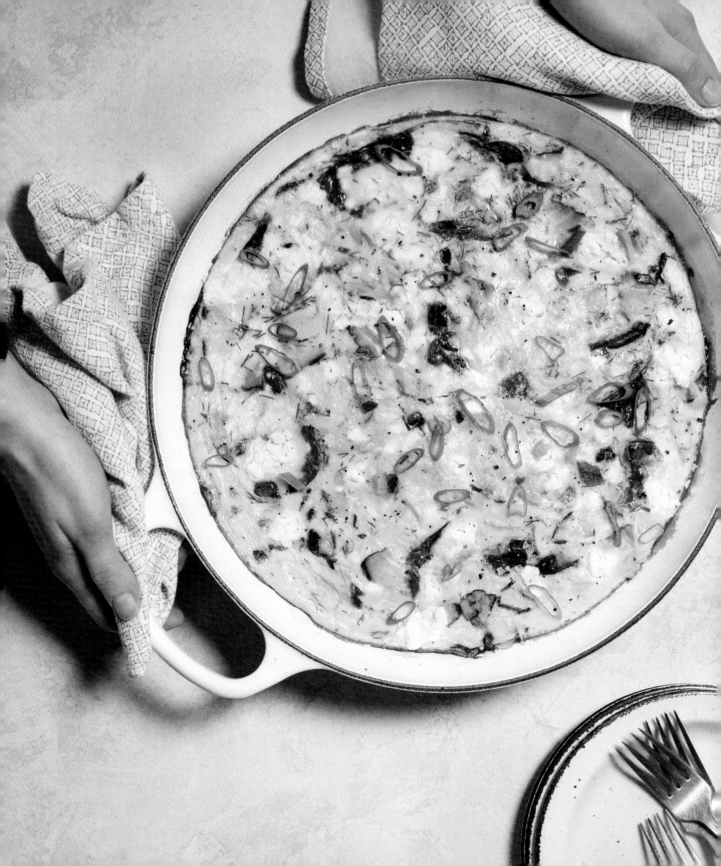

smoked salmon frittata with goat cheese

Prep Time: **10 minutes** | Cook Time: **30 minutes** | Total Time: **40 minutes** | Makes **8 servings**

GF
GrF
NF

2 teaspoons avocado oil or extra-virgin olive oil
1 bunch green onions, trimmed and thinly sliced
2 garlic cloves, minced
5 ounces loosely packed baby spinach (5 cups)
12 large eggs
½ cup milk of choice
2 tablespoons chopped fresh dill (or 2 teaspoons dried dill)
¼ teaspoon ground black pepper
Pinch of fine salt
8 ounces smoked salmon, skin removed and discarded, roughly chopped
4 ounces soft goat cheese, crumbled

Tips from the Dietitians

If you do not have a large oven-safe skillet, you can cook the vegetables in a medium skillet of any kind and then transfer them to a 3- to 4-quart greased casserole dish, spreading out the spinach. Proceed with topping the spinach evenly with the salmon and pouring the egg mixture over the spinach. Then top evenly with the goat cheese. Bake according to recipe directions.

The addition of smoked salmon and creamy goat cheese elevates an everyday frittata to something extraordinary and worthy of your most special occasions. Whether it's a brunch for Mother's Day, a baby shower, or a low-key weekend gathering with friends, when you want to pull out all the stops we know you'll appreciate the fact that it takes so little work to get such impressive results. Make your brunch even more special by adding Oven-Baked French Toast Casserole (page 39), yogurt topped with Your Go-To Granola (page 21), or Berry or Peachy Green Smoothies (page 41).

Preheat the oven to 375°F.

Place a large oven-safe skillet over medium-high heat. If you do not have a large oven-safe skillet, see Tips. When the skillet is hot, add the avocado oil and swirl to coat. Add the green onions and garlic and cook, stirring occasionally, until fragrant, 2 to 3 minutes. Add the spinach and cook, stirring occasionally, until wilted, about 2 minutes.

Whisk the eggs and milk in a large bowl, then stir in the dill, pepper, and the salt.

Decrease the heat slightly under the skillet. Spread out the spinach and top evenly with the salmon. Pour the egg mixture over the top. Then top evenly with the goat cheese. Increase the heat slightly and cook, undisturbed, until the sides begin to set, 3 to 4 minutes.

Transfer to the oven and bake for 17 to 20 minutes, or until the center of the frittata is firm. Remove from the oven and let it set for 5 minutes before serving.

Store leftovers in an airtight container in the refrigerator for up to 4 days.

Nutrition Info: (Serving size: ⅛ recipe) 184 calories, 12g total fat, 5g saturated fat, 367mg sodium, 2g carbs, 1g sugar, 1g fiber, 16g protein

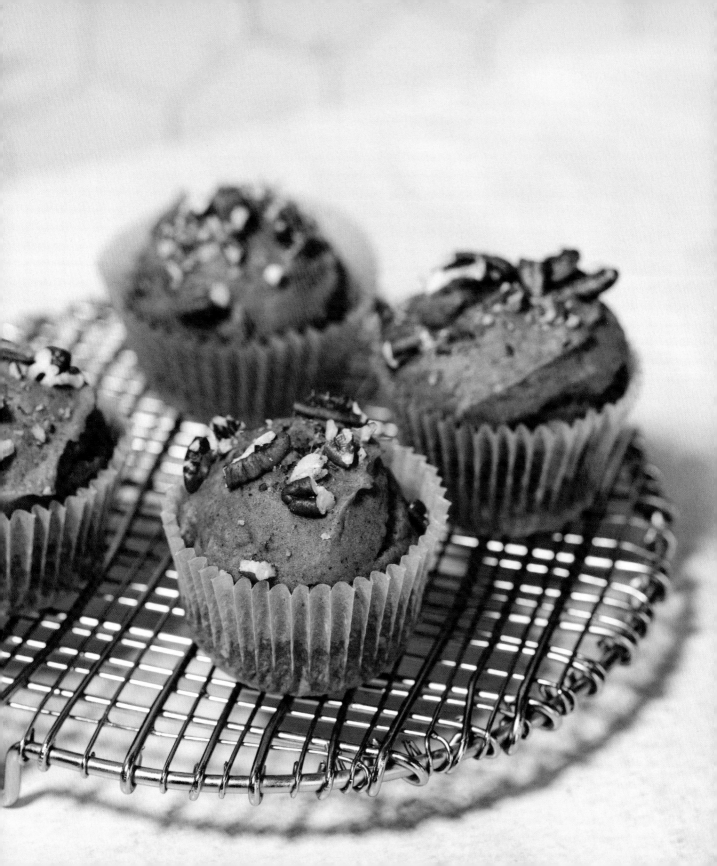

pumpkin muffins with toasted pecans

Prep time: **15 minutes** | Cook time: **15 minutes** | Total time: **30 minutes** | Makes: **12 muffins**

GF

DF

VEG

NFO

Nonstick cooking spray
½ cup chopped pecans, divided (omit for nut-free)
1½ cups gluten-free all-purpose flour blend
2 teaspoons pumpkin pie spice
1 teaspoon baking soda
½ teaspoon ground cinnamon
¼ teaspoon fine salt
1 cup canned pumpkin puree (not pumpkin pie filling)
⅓ cup packed brown sugar (light or dark)
2 large eggs
¼ cup avocado oil or extra-virgin olive oil
3 tablespoons pure maple syrup
2 teaspoons pure vanilla extract

Tips from the Dietitians
Mix in a handful of chocolate chips with, or in place of, the pecans to make the most delicious pumpkin chocolate chip muffins!

Soft, tender, and made with less sugar than most store-bought muffins, these pumpkin muffins are calling your name! They're studded with toasted pecans and can be enjoyed as part of breakfast, an afternoon snack, or a tasty treat with a cup of coffee or tea. Feel free to double this recipe and tuck some away in the freezer for later.

Preheat the oven to 375°F. Line a 12-cup muffin tin with paper liners. Lightly spray each liner with cooking spray and set aside.

Place a small skillet over medium-low heat. Add the pecans and cook, stirring occasionally until the pecans give off a toasted aroma, 7 to 8 minutes. Remove from the heat and transfer the pecans to a plate to cool.

In a large bowl, combine the flour, pumpkin pie spice, baking soda, cinnamon, and salt, and mix well.

In a medium bowl, combine the pumpkin puree, brown sugar, eggs, avocado oil, maple syrup, and vanilla, and to stir to mix well. Add the wet ingredients to the dry ingredients along with ⅓ cup of the cooled pecans and stir until everything is combined.

Transfer the batter to the prepared muffin tin, filling each well about halfway. Sprinkle the remaining pecans over the tops of the muffins.

Bake for 15 to 18 minutes, or until a toothpick inserted in the center of a muffin comes out clean.

Remove the pan from the oven and let cool for 5 to 10 minutes on a wire rack, then transfer each muffin to the wire rack to cool.

Store in an airtight container or large zip-top bag in the refrigerator for up to 1 week or in the freezer for up to 3 months.

Nutrition Info: (Serving size: 1 muffin) 195 calories, 8g total fat, 1g saturated fat, 95mg sodium, 28g carbs, 10g sugar, 1g fiber, 3g protein

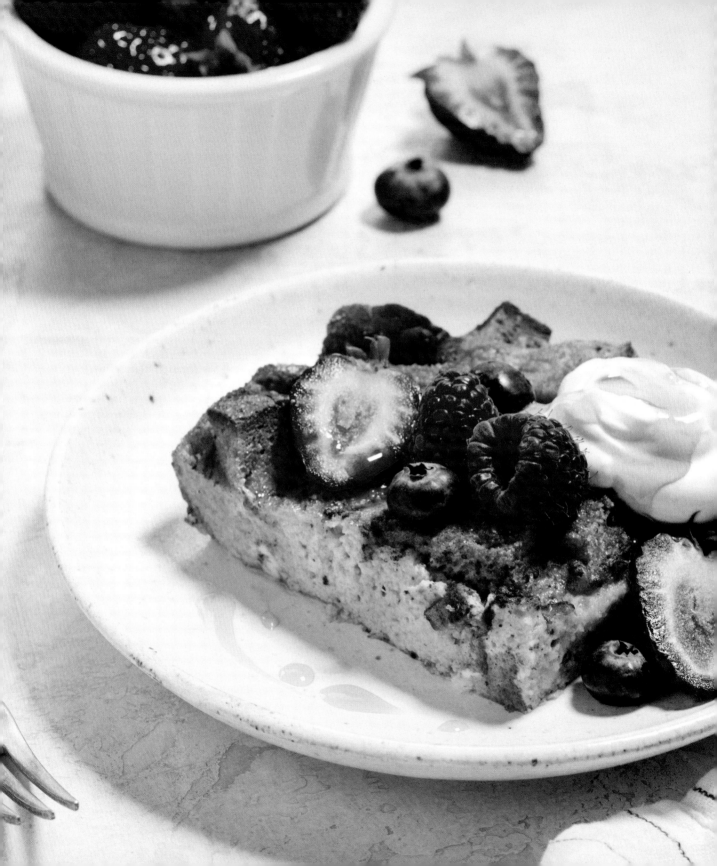

oven-baked french toast casserole

Prep Time: **15 minutes** | Cook Time: **45 minutes** | Total Time: **1 hour, plus 5 minutes for cooling** | Makes **6**

GF
DFO
VEG
NF

Butter (or nonstick cooking spray, for dairy-free), for greasing
10 to 12 ounces gluten-free bread of choice, cut into ¾-inch cubes (6 cups)
6 large eggs
2 cups milk (or nondairy milk, for dairy-free)
2 tablespoons pure maple syrup
2 teaspoons pure vanilla extract
1½ teaspoons ground cinnamon, divided
Pinch of ground nutmeg
1 tablespoon sugar

Optional toppings:
Yogurt or nondairy whipped topping, fresh fruit and/or pure maple syrup

This breakfast casserole, reminiscent of bread pudding, spares you from having to stand over the stove and dip, cook, and flip just a few slices of French toast at a time. It's a great dish to serve at holiday brunches or for a lazy weekend breakfast. It's also a good way to stretch your grocery bill, since you can make the casserole with leftover bits of bread—any type works, even dinner rolls or buns.

Preheat the oven to 350°F. Grease a 9×9-inch baking dish generously with butter or cooking spray, add the bread, and set aside.

In a medium bowl, whisk the eggs, milk, maple syrup, vanilla, 1 teaspoon of the cinnamon, and the nutmeg. Pour over the bread, carefully pressing down with a rubber spatula to saturate the bread.

In a small bowl, combine the sugar with the remaining ½ teaspoon cinnamon. Sprinkle over the casserole.

Bake for about 45 minutes, or until the top of the casserole is golden brown and a toothpick inserted into the center comes out clean.

Remove the baking dish from the oven and allow the casserole to cool for 5 minutes, then cut into 6 pieces.

Serve topped with yogurt or whipped topping, fruit, and/or maple syrup, if desired. Store leftovers in an airtight container in the refrigerator for up to 4 days.

Tips from the Dietitians
This is a great way to use up stale bread and cut down on kitchen waste. We keep a zip-top bag in the freezer to collect the heels of bread, leftover hamburger buns, dinner rolls, etc., then make a batch of this French toast when there's enough for six cups of bread cubes.

Nutrition Info: (Serving size: ⅙ of recipe) 236 calories, 7g total fat, 3g saturated fat, 301mg sodium, 33g carbs, 11g sugar, 3g fiber, 9g protein

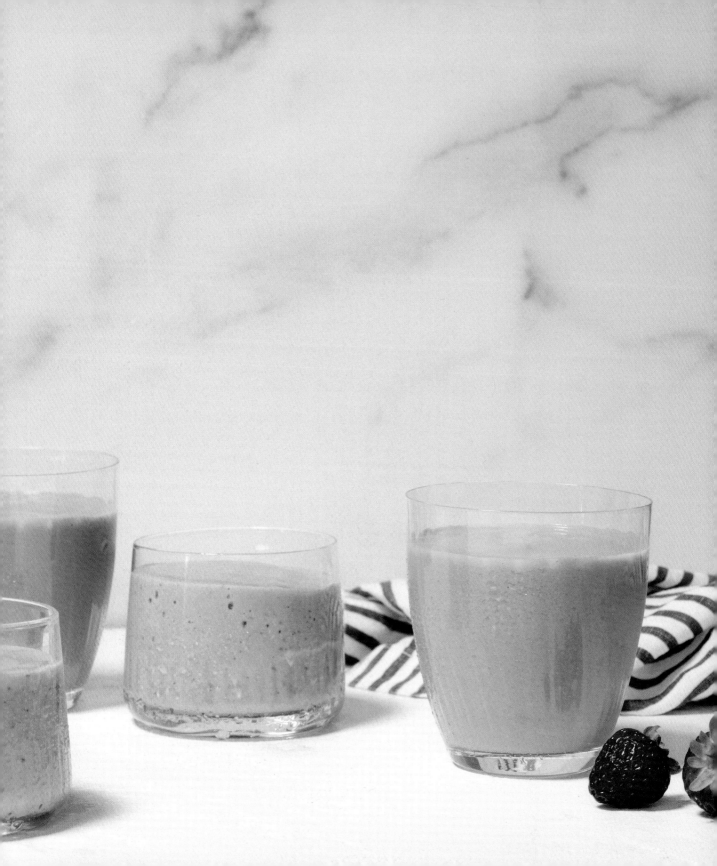

berry or peachy green smoothies

Prep Time: **5 minutes** | Total Time: **5 minutes** | Makes **2 servings**

GF

GrF

DFO

EF

VEG

VO

NF

NAS

1½ cups frozen mixed berries or sliced peaches

½ cup frozen cauliflower rice or florets

1 small banana

1 cup loosely packed baby spinach

½ avocado, peeled or scooped from the skin

¾ cup milk (or nondairy milk, for dairy-free and vegan), plus more for a thinner consistency

½ cup Greek plain yogurt or additional milk of choice (see Tips)

Optional Smoothie Nutrition Boosters

1 tablespoon chia seeds, flaxseed, or hemp hearts

1 tablespoon cacao nibs or powder

1 to 2 Brazil nuts (for selenium)

3 to 5 walnut halves (for omega-3 fatty acids)

1 scoop of your favorite protein powder (may need to add more liquid to blend)

Here are two delicious smoothie options to start your day off right. Choose between frozen mixed berries or peaches. The smoothies are packed with real food ingredients including naturally sweet fruits, leafy greens, cauliflower, and a healthy dose of fat from avocado. Perfect to drink on the go, and kid friendly, too! Stacie whips up a little smoothie nearly every morning for her daughter, who slurps it down in a matter of minutes. Add an optional nutrition booster (or two), if desired.

Add the berries, cauliflower, banana, spinach, avocado, milk, and yogurt, plus one or two of the nutrition boosters, if desired, to a blender. Turn the blender on low and gradually increase the speed. Blend until smooth.

For a thinner consistency, blend in more milk of your choice a little at a time until you reach your desired consistency.

Tips from the Dietitians

For a dairy-free and vegan-friendly smoothie, substitute a nondairy yogurt for the Greek yogurt, or omit the yogurt and add 1¼ cups nondairy milk of choice instead of ¾ cup.

For a nut-free option, choose a non nut-based milk, like oat milk.

Feel free to use your frozen fruit of choice instead of the mixed berries or peaches.

As fresh fruits, greens, or avocados you have on hand near the end of their shelf life, simply place them in a zip-top bag and store in the freezer to use in future smoothies.

For the Berry Green Smoothies
Nutrition Info: (Serving size: 1½ cups) 148 calories, 9g total fat, 3g saturated fat, 80mg sodium, 23g carbs, 17g sugar, 5g fiber, 11g protein

For the Peachy Green Smoothies
Nutrition Info: (Serving size: 1½ cups) 140 calories, 8g total fat, 3g saturated fat, 80mg sodium, 21g carbs, 17g sugar, 4g fiber, 11g protein

salads & sides

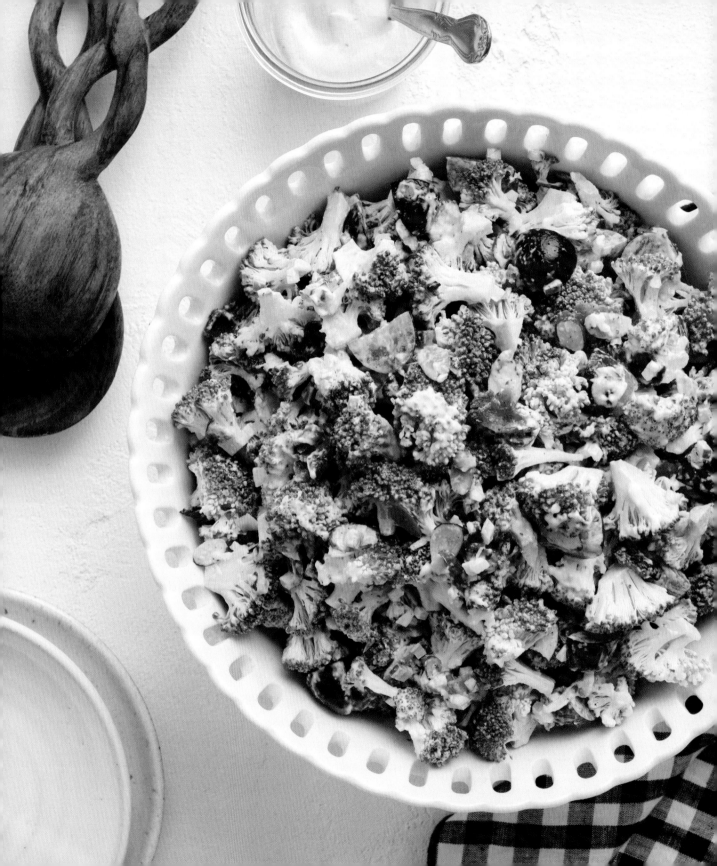

the best broccoli salad

Prep Time: **25 minutes** | Total Time: **25 minutes** | Makes **8 servings**

GF
GrF
DF
EFO
NFO
NAS

FOR THE BROCCOLI MIXTURE
¼ cup sliced or slivered almonds (omit for nut-free; see Tips)
4 bacon slices (4 ounces; see Tips)
1 large head broccoli (about 1 pound), trimmed and cut into bite-size florets (5 to 5½ cups)
1 cup seedless red grapes, halved
¼ cup finely diced red onion

FOR THE DRESSING
½ cup mayonnaise (or vegan mayonnaise for egg-free; see Tips)
3 tablespoons apple cider vinegar
½ teaspoon garlic powder
½ teaspoon fine salt
Pinch of ground black pepper

Tips from the Dietitians
If you're planning to prepare this salad ahead to take to a potluck or party, reserve the chopped bacon and toasted almonds to add later, then store the dressing and salad in separate containers in the refrigerator for up to 3 days. Make the salad up to 30 minutes before serving.

If you're looking to avoid added sugars, use bacon and mayonnaise made without sugar.

To make this nut-free, substitute sunflower seeds for the almonds.

When Jessica was growing up, her grandma made broccoli salad for weekends at the family cabin in northern Minnesota. Jessica and her cousins nicknamed the dish "Wood Tick Salad" because it had sunflower seeds, which bore a striking resemblance to the pesky little wood ticks that are so abundant in the summer in that area. This broccoli salad is a healthy remake of that family favorite, which was heavy on the mayo and white sugar. To lighten it up, we added just enough mayo to keep it creamy, left out the added sugar, and swapped fresh red grapes for the raisins (because Jessica would just pick those out anyway). She makes the salad now with almonds, but for a nut-free option, you can replace the almonds with sunflower seeds.

Prepare the broccoli mixture: Place a small skillet over medium heat. When hot, add the almonds and cook, stirring often, until they are golden and give off a toasted aroma, 6 to 8 minutes. Transfer the almonds to a plate to cool.

Wipe the skillet clean and place it over medium-high heat. When hot, add the bacon and cook until crisp, 2 to 3 minutes per side. Remove the bacon to a paper towel–lined plate. Let cool, then roughly chop and set aside.

In a large bowl, combine the broccoli, grapes, onion, almonds, and bacon. Set aside.

Make the dressing: In a small bowl, combine the mayonnaise, vinegar, garlic powder, salt, and black pepper. Whisk to combine.

Pour the dressing over the broccoli mixture and stir gently to combine and serve (see Tips).

Store leftovers in an airtight container in the refrigerator for up to 3 days.

Nutrition Info: (Serving size: ¾ cup) 154 calories, 13g total fat, 2g saturated fat, 327mg sodium, 7g carbs, 3g sugar, 2g fiber, 4g protein

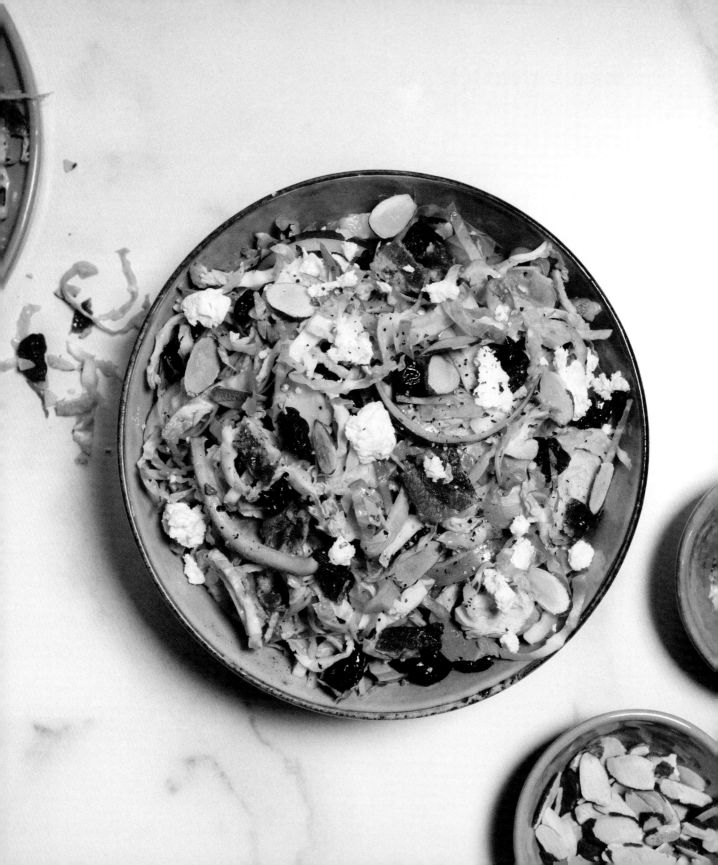

shredded brussels sprouts salad with citrus vinaigrette

GF GrF DFO EF NFO

Prep Time: **20 minutes** | Cook Time: **15 minutes** | Total Time: **35 minutes** | Make **14 servings**

FOR THE BRUSSELS SPROUTS MIXTURE
⅔ cup sliced or slivered almonds (omit for nut-free; see Tips)
6 bacon slices (6 ounces)
24 ounces Brussels sprouts, trimmed and shredded (see Tips)
½ medium red onion, thinly sliced
⅔ cup dried cranberries or dried cherries
4 ounces soft goat cheese, crumbled (omit for dairy-free)

FOR THE CITRUS VINAIGRETTE
½ cup avocado oil or extra-virgin olive oil
1 teaspoon grated orange zest
⅓ cup fresh orange juice (1 medium orange)
3 tablespoons fresh lemon juice (1 medium lemon)
1 small shallot, minced
2 teaspoons pure maple syrup
2 teaspoons fresh thyme leaves (or ½ teaspoon dried thyme)
1 teaspoon Dijon mustard
Fine salt and ground black pepper

Tips from the Dietitians
For the Brussels sprouts, use two 10-ounce bags of pre-shredded or, if shredding your own, use the shredding blade of a food processor.

To make this nut-free, substitute sunflower seeds for the almonds.

Hands down, this is one of Stacie's favorite salads to make year-round! Shredded Brussels sprouts are the base for this scrumptious salad. They're hearty enough to stand up to all the other textures and flavors: toasted almonds, tart dried cherries (or cranberries), smoky, crisp bacon, and crumbled goat cheese. A bright citrus vinaigrette ties together all of the flavors. This is a salad you'll most definitely want to bring to all of your family gatherings, backyard barbecues, picnics, and potlucks.

Prepare the Brussels sprouts mixture: Place a small skillet over medium heat. When hot, add the almonds and cook, stirring often, until they are golden and give off a toasted aroma, 6 to 8 minutes. Transfer the almonds to a plate to cool.

Wipe the skillet clean and place it over medium-high heat. When hot, add the bacon and cook until crisp, 2 to 3 minutes per side. Remove the bacon to a paper towel–lined plate. Let cool, then roughly chop and set aside.

In a large bowl, combine the Brussels sprouts, onion, cranberries, bacon, and almonds.

Make the citrus vinaigrette: In a small bowl, combine the avocado oil, orange zest, orange juice, lemon juice, shallot, maple syrup, thyme, and mustard. Whisk well to emulsify. Add salt and pepper to taste.

Pour the vinaigrette over the Brussels sprouts mixture just before serving and toss until all of the ingredients are well coated. Add the goat cheese and toss gently to mix.

Store leftovers in an airtight container in the refrigerator for up to 3 days.

Nutrition Info: (Serving size: ¾ cup) 180 calories, 14g total fat, 3g saturated fat, 121mg sodium, 11g carbs, 6g sugar, 2g fiber, 5g protein

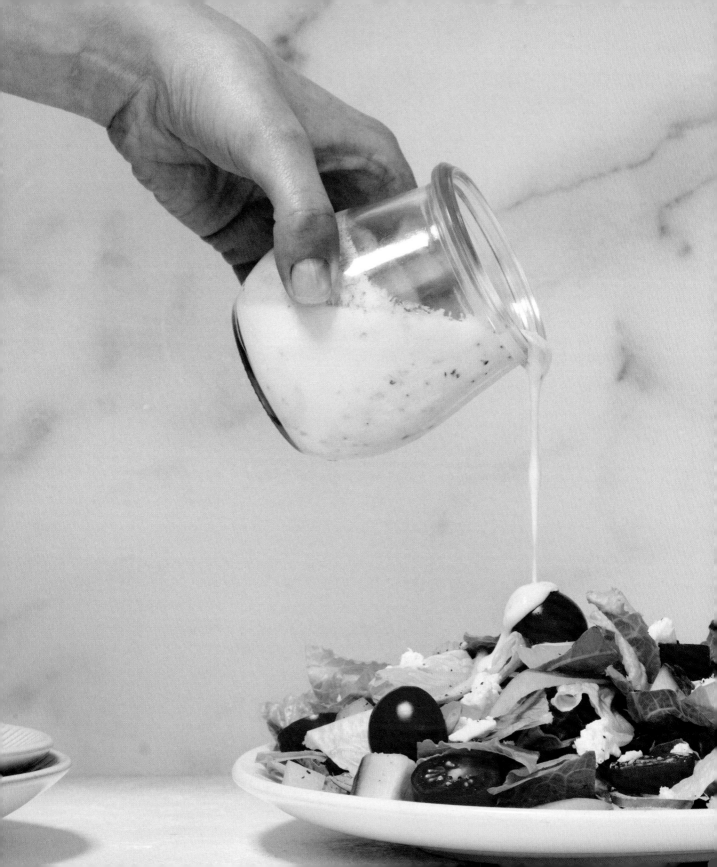

greek chopped salad

Prep Time: **20 minutes** | Total Time: **20 minutes** | Makes **4 servings**

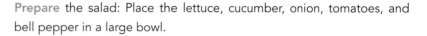

FOR THE SALAD

6 cups chopped romaine lettuce

1 English cucumber, diced
   (3 cups)

¼ medium red onion, very thinly
   sliced (⅓ cup)

1 cup grape tomatoes, halved
   (6 ounces)

1 small yellow bell pepper, diced
   (1 cup)

FOR THE DRESSING

½ cup crumbled feta cheese

⅓ cup Greek Vinaigrette and
   Marinade (page 258)

¼ cup plain Greek yogurt

The beauty of this chopped salad is that it's low-fuss but big on flavor. It satisfies our desire for crisp and crunchy with bites of cool cucumber, bell pepper, and romaine lettuce all dressed up in a creamy yogurt and feta dressing. It's the perfect no-cook, keep-the-kitchen-cool side salad for your favorite grilled protein or rotisserie chicken.

Prepare the salad: Place the lettuce, cucumber, onion, tomatoes, and bell pepper in a large bowl.

Make the dressing: In a food processor or blender, combine the feta, vinaigrette, and yogurt. Pulse until the dressing is mostly smooth but still slightly chunky, 5 to 10 times.

Pour the dressing over the salad and toss to combine (see Tips).

Store leftovers in separate airtight containers in the refrigerator for up to 3 days.

Tips from the Dietitians

If you're planning to prepare this salad ahead, store the dressing and salad in separate airtight containers in the refrigerator until ready to serve, for up to 3 days. If the dressing separates in the refrigerator, give it a good shake or stir before using.

Nutrition Info: (Serving size: 2 cups) 218 calories, 17g total fat, 5g saturated fat, 404mg sodium, 11g carbs, 7g sugar, 2g fiber, 7g protein

GF
GrF
EF
VEG
NF
NAS

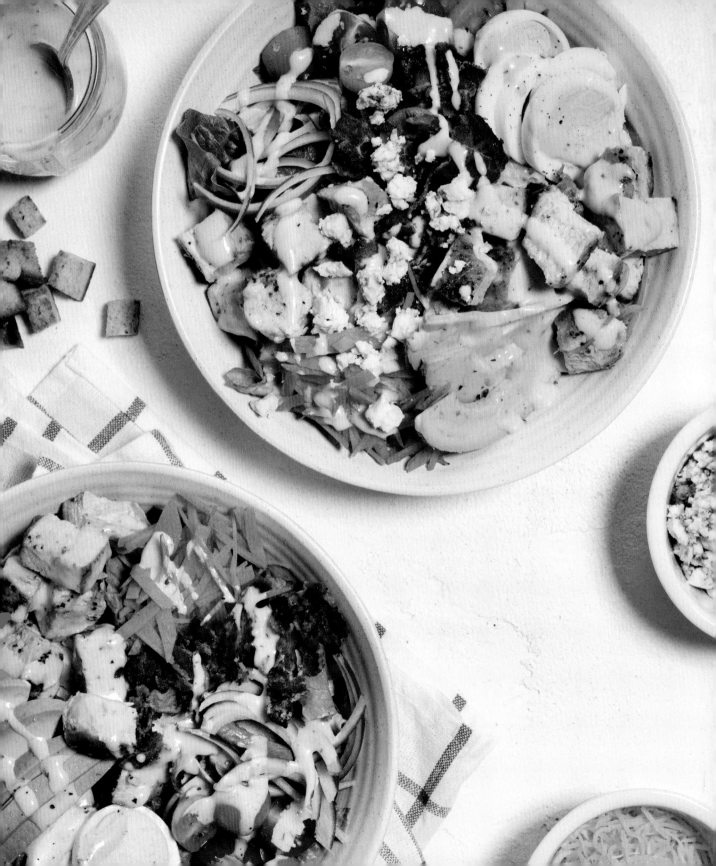

big cobb salad for two

Prep Time: **30 minutes** | Cook Time: **20 minutes** | Total Time: **50 minutes** | Makes **2 main-course servings**

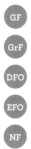

2 bacon slices (2 ounces)
¼ teaspoon garlic powder
¼ teaspoon onion powder
¼ teaspoon fine salt
⅛ teaspoon ground black pepper
1 large boneless, skinless chicken breast (6 to 8 ounces), patted dry
2 teaspoons avocado oil or extra-virgin olive oil
4 cups chopped romaine lettuce
⅔ cup grape tomatoes, halved
½ cup thinly sliced red onion
½ cup shredded carrots
½ medium avocado, sliced
¼ cup shredded cheddar cheese or crumbled blue cheese (omit for dairy-free)
2 Easy-Peel Hard-Boiled Eggs (page 211), sliced (omit for egg-free)
4 tablespoons Honey Mustard Dressing and Dipping Sauce (page 259)

Optional topping:
Garlic-Herb Croutons (page 269)

This salad truly has it all: juicy chicken, crisp bacon, creamy avocado, cheese, hard-boiled eggs, and, oh yeah, plenty of veggies, too. It's dressed in our oh-so-creamy honey mustard dressing, and if you want to top it with a few homemade garlic-herb croutons, go right ahead. Not a salad lover? Well, you have to give us a chance here. This is more than just a salad, it's a new and flavorful experience that will get you to love salad. Every forkful will leave your belly and your taste buds pleasantly satisfied.

Place a medium skillet over medium-high heat. When hot, add the bacon and cook until crisp, 2 to 3 minutes per side. Remove the bacon to a paper towel–lined plate. Let cool, then roughly chop and set aside.

In a small bowl, mix the garlic powder, onion powder, salt, and pepper. Sprinkle both sides of the chicken with this seasoning mix.

Place a grill pan over medium-high heat. When hot, brush it with the avocado oil. Add the chicken and cook on one side, undisturbed, until lightly browned, 8 to 10 minutes. Flip and cook, undisturbed, until an instant-read thermometer registers 165°F in the center of the breast, 8 to 10 minutes. Transfer the chicken to a cutting board and let rest for 5 to 10 minutes while you prepare the salads.

Divide the lettuce between two large salad bowls. Top each bowl with half of the tomatoes, onion, carrots, bacon, avocado, cheese, and eggs. Slice or dice the chicken, and divide it between the two salads.

Drizzle the salads with Honey Mustard Dressing, then top each with a few Garlic-Herb Croutons, if desired.

Store leftover salad and dressing separately in airtight containers in the refrigerator for up to 2 days.

Nutrition Info: (Serving size: 1 salad with 2 tablespoons dressing and without the croutons) 547 calories, 37g total fat, 9g saturated fat, 1,104mg sodium, 17g carbs, 9g sugar, 5g fiber, 33g protein

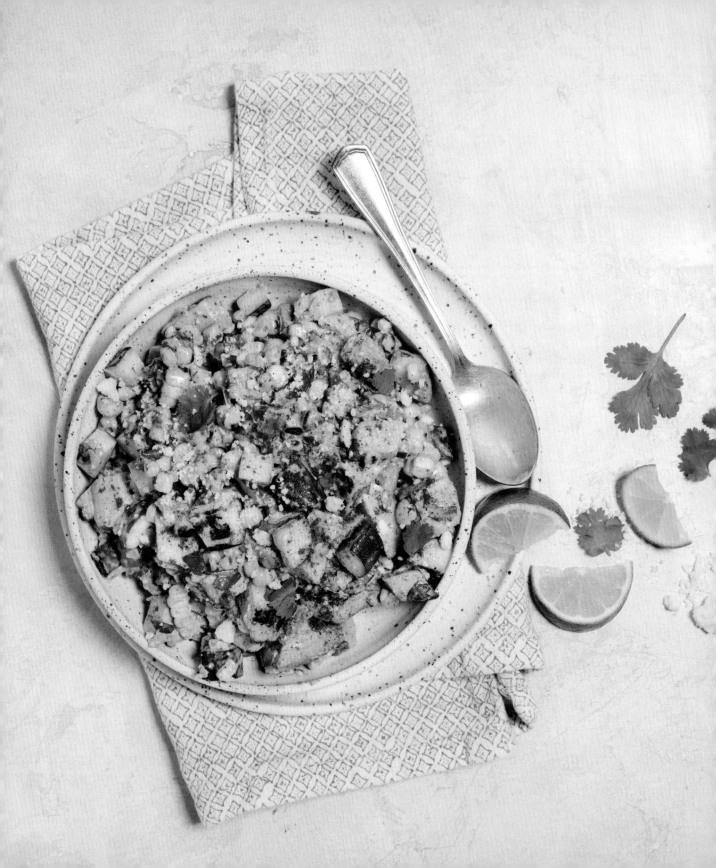

mexican street corn–style salad

Prep Time: **15 minutes** | Cook Time: **25 minutes** | Total Time: **40 minutes** | Makes **8 servings**

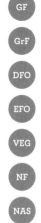

FOR THE CORN SALAD

Nonstick cooking spray, if using a grill pan

2 large ears sweet corn, husk removed

2 medium zucchini, cut lengthwise into ½-inch-thick slices

1 tablespoon avocado oil or extra-virgin olive oil

Fine salt and ground black pepper

1 medium avocado, diced

½ cup loosely packed fresh cilantro leaves, roughly chopped

⅓ cup crumbled cotija cheese (1½ ounces; omit for dairy-free)

¼ cup finely diced red onion

FOR THE DRESSING

2 tablespoons mayonnaise (use vegan mayonnaise, for egg-free; see Tips)

1 teaspoon grated lime zest (1 small lime)

1½ tablespoons fresh lime juice (from the zested lime)

1¼ teaspoons chili powder

Fine salt and ground black pepper

This salad was inspired by *elote*, or Mexican street corn. Street vendors grill sweet ears of corn until the kernels are lightly charred and tender. They slather the corn with a mixture of creamy mayonnaise and tart lime juice, then sprinkle them with chili powder, finely minced cilantro, and salty cotija cheese. Whenever Jessica's daughters spot a roadside vendor or lunch cart selling *elote*, they beg to stop. The combination of sweet, creamy, spicy, and tart is absolutely addictive. We've combined all of those flavors in this corn salad and added grilled zucchini and fresh avocado for our own twist that makes it hard to stop eating. Pair it with your favorite Mexican-inspired dishes, a simple grilled salmon fillet, steak, or chicken breast, or just scoop it up with your favorite tortilla chips.

For the corn salad: Preheat a grill to medium-high heat (425°F), and prepare it for direct and indirect heat. Alternatively, spray a large grill pan with cooking spray and preheat it over medium-high heat.

Brush the corn and zucchini with the avocado oil, and sprinkle with salt and pepper.

Place the corn on the grill grates over direct heat (or the grill pan) and grill, turning occasionally, until the corn is lightly charred all over, about 10 minutes. Move the corn to indirect heat (or the cooler parts of the grill pan) and continue cooking, turning occasionally, until the corn is tender, about 10 minutes.

Add the zucchini to the grill grates over indirect heat (or the cooler parts of the grill pan) and grill, flipping halfway through, until crisp-tender and lightly grill-marked, 10 to 12 minutes.

Transfer the corn and zucchini to a plate and allow to cool while you make the dressing.

Continued on the next page

In a small bowl, combine the mayonnaise, lime zest and juice, and chili powder. Whisk well. Add salt and pepper to taste.

Once the vegetables are cool, cut the corn kernels from the cobs and dice the zucchini into ½-inch pieces. Transfer both to a large bowl. Add the avocado, cilantro, cotija cheese, and onion.

Pour the dressing over the corn salad and toss gently to coat. Serve right away.

Store leftovers in an airtight container in the refrigerator for up to 3 days.

Tips from the Dietitians

If you're looking to avoid added sugars, use mayonnaise that is made without sugar.

Nutrition Info: (Serving size: ⅔ cup) 113 calories, 8g total fat, 2g saturated fat, 102mg sodium, 8g carbs, 1g sugar, 2g fiber, 2g protein

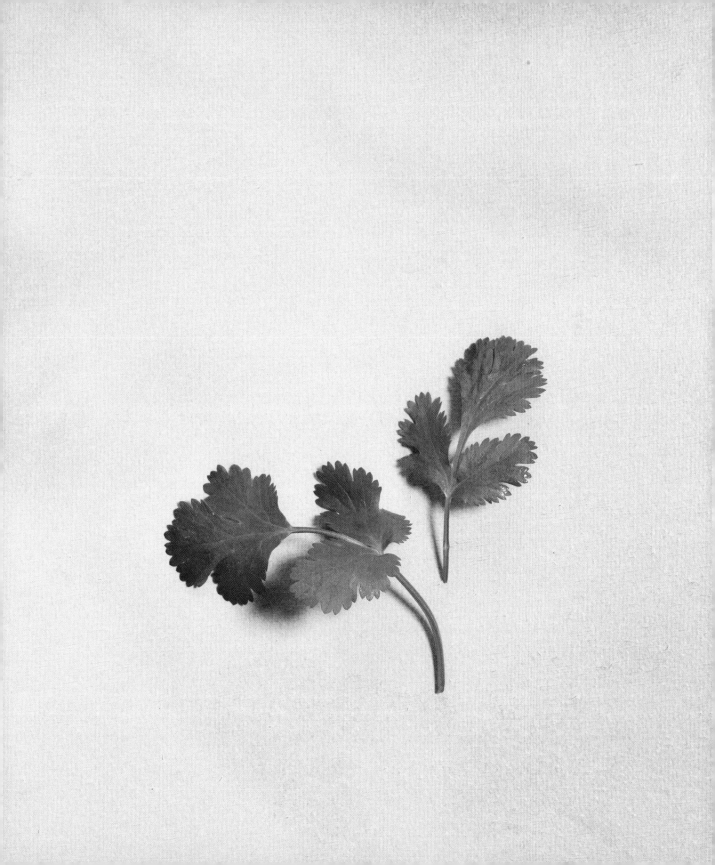

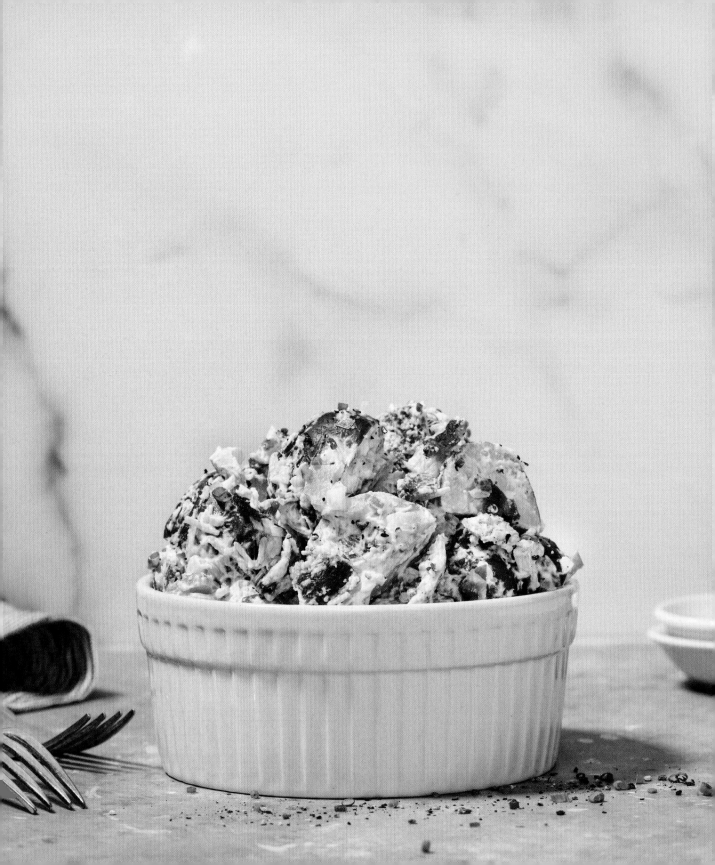

loaded baked potato salad

Prep Time: **15 minutes** | Cook Time: **25 minutes, plus 15 minutes for cooling** | Total Time: **55 minutes** | Makes **4 servings**

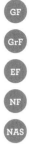

1 pound baby red potatoes, scrubbed clean and cut into ¾-inch pieces

Fine salt and ground black pepper

4 bacon slices (4 ounces; see Tips)

½ cup sour cream

2 tablespoons apple cider vinegar

½ teaspoon garlic powder

2 celery stalks, thinly sliced (½ cup)

⅓ cup shredded cheddar cheese

2 tablespoons finely chopped red onion

2 tablespoons chopped fresh chives (or 2 teaspoons dried chives)

Tips from the Dietitians

If you're looking to avoid added sugars, use bacon that is made without sugar.

This salad takes its inspiration from those loaded baked potatoes that were made popular by steakhouses and supper clubs of yesteryear. It's got everything you love in a baked potato—smoky bacon, fragrant chives, tangy sour cream, and savory cheddar cheese—all without turning on the oven. Watch this salad become the hit of every backyard barbecue, potluck, or family gathering. It'll go quick, so don't be afraid to make a double batch and save some for yourself. You won't regret it!

Place the potatoes in a medium saucepan. Add enough water to cover the potatoes by 1 to 2 inches and generously salt the water. Bring to a boil, then decrease the heat slightly to prevent the water from boiling over. Cook the potatoes until tender when pierced with a fork, 15 to 20 minutes.

Drain the potatoes, transfer them to a medium bowl, and refrigerate until cooled to room temperature, about 20 minutes.

Meanwhile, place a medium skillet over medium-high heat. When hot, add the bacon and cook until crisp, 2 to 3 minutes per side. Remove the bacon to a paper towel–lined plate. Let cool, then roughly chop and set aside.

In a small bowl, combine the sour cream, vinegar, and garlic powder. Whisk well. Add salt and pepper to taste. Set aside.

Remove the cooled potatoes from the refrigerator. To the same bowl, add the celery, cheddar, onion, chives, and bacon.

Pour the dressing over the potatoes and stir gently to combine. Serve right away or refrigerate until ready to serve.

Store leftovers in an airtight container in the refrigerator for up to 4 days.

Nutrition Info: (Serving size: ¾ cup) 210 calories, 11g total fat, 6g saturated fat, 249mg sodium, 20g carbs, 5g sugar, 2g fiber, 9g protein

cilantro-lime slaw

Prep Time: **15 minutes** | Total Time: **15 minutes** | Makes **4 servings**

FOR THE SLAW

4 cups thinly sliced red cabbage
   or bagged coleslaw mix
   (9 to 10 ounces)
½ cup loosely packed fresh
   cilantro leaves, roughly
   chopped

FOR THE DRESSING

1 tablespoon avocado oil or extra-
   virgin olive oil
1 tablespoon apple cider vinegar
1 tablespoon fresh lime juice
   (½ medium lime)
1 teaspoon honey (or agave
   nectar, for vegan; omit for no
   sugar added)
¼ teaspoon ground cumin
¼ teaspoon fine salt
Pinch of chipotle powder or
   cayenne pepper (optional)

This simple yet spectacular slaw features one of our favorite long-storing and antioxidant-packed vegetables. The humble cabbage (or bagged coleslaw mix, if you need a shortcut) gets a lift from a lightly sweet, tangy, and slightly earthy dressing. It's our go-to side dish whenever tacos, burrito bowls, or Turkey Taco Casserole (page 109) are on the menu, or whenever you want to add a little crunch and color to a meal.

Prepare the slaw: Combine the cabbage and cilantro in a medium bowl. Set aside.

Make the dressing: In a small bowl, combine the avocado oil, vinegar, lime juice, honey, cumin, salt, and chipotle powder, if using. Whisk well to emulsify.

Pour the dressing over the slaw and toss to combine (see Tips).

Store leftovers in an airtight container in the refrigerator for up to 3 days.

Tips from the Dietitians

If you're planning to prepare this slaw ahead to take to a potluck or party, or as part of a meal prep, store the dressing and slaw in separate containers in the refrigerator until ready to use. Toss everything together up to 30 minutes before serving.

Nutrition Info: (Serving size: ⅔ cup) 65 calories, 4g total fat, 0g saturated fat, 173mg sodium, 8g carbs, 5g sugar, 2g fiber, 1g protein

every occasion coleslaw

Prep Time: **10 minutes** | Total Time: **10 minutes, plus 15 minutes for resting** | Makes **6 servings**

GF
GrF
DF
EFO
VEG
VO
NF
NAS

4 cups bagged coleslaw mix
(9 to 10 ounces) or thinly sliced
cabbage
⅓ cup mayonnaise (or vegan
mayonnaise, for egg-free and
vegan; see Tips)
3 tablespoons apple cider vinegar
1 teaspoon honey (or agave
nectar, for vegan; omit for no
added sugar)
¼ teaspoon garlic powder
Fine salt and ground black pepper

We can think of very few meals that don't benefit from the addition of creamy coleslaw. This one takes less than 5 minutes to make when you start with a bag of coleslaw mix. The dressing has just the right amount of tang and is made with less mayo to create a lighter version of this popular cabbage salad. We love to scoop it on top of Shredded Barbecue Beef–Stuffed Sweet Potatoes (page 135) and Instant Pot Pulled Pork (page 155), but of course it's also great served on the side. This slaw is also the perfect pairing for Easier-Than-Ever Slow Cooker Baby Back Ribs (page 158), Sheet Pan Fish-and-Chips with Tartar Sauce (page 167), and Crispy Baked Chicken Nuggets (page 85).

Place the coleslaw mix in a medium bowl.

In a small bowl, combine the mayonnaise, vinegar, honey, and garlic powder. Whisk well to combine. Add salt and pepper to taste.

Pour the dressing over the coleslaw mix and toss to combine. Let stand for 15 minutes before serving.

Store leftovers in an airtight container in the refrigerator for up to 3 days.

> **Tips from the Dietitians**
> If you're looking to avoid added sugars, use mayonnaise that is made without sugar.

Nutrition Info: (Serving size: ¾ cup) 89 calories, 9g total fat, 1g saturated fat, 93mg sodium, 2g carbs, 1g sugar, 1g fiber, 1g protein

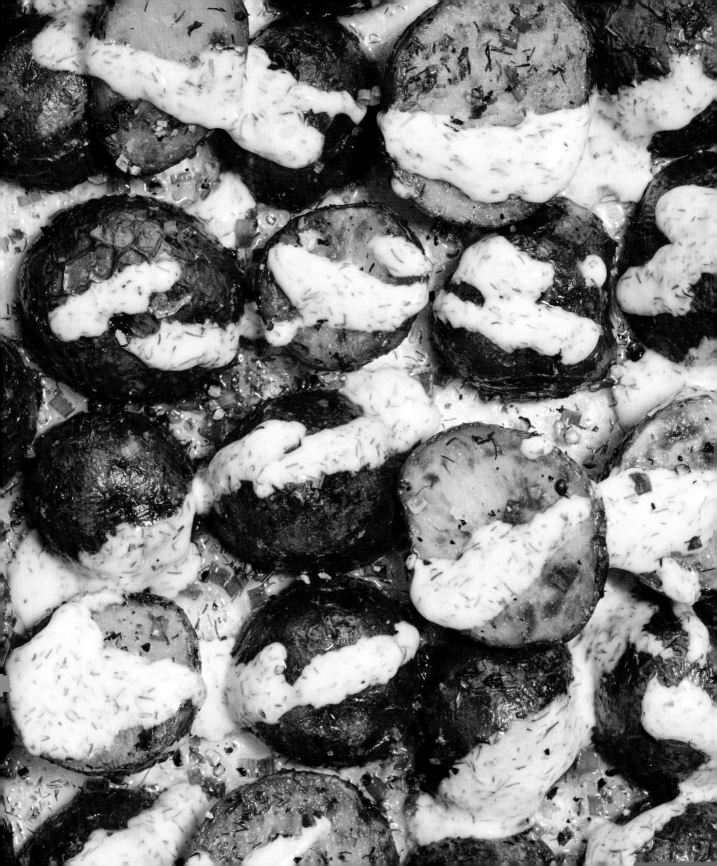

ranch roasted potatoes

Prep Time: **15 minutes** | Cook Time: **40 minutes** | Total Time: **55 minutes** | Makes **6 servings**

GF

GrF

DFO

EF

VEG

VO

NF

NAS

1½ pounds baby red potatoes, scrubbed clean and halved lengthwise

¼ cup (4 tablespoons) unsalted butter, melted (or scant ¼ cup avocado oil or extra-virgin olive oil, for dairy-free and vegan)

1½ tablespoons Ranch Seasoning Mix (page 257)

¼ teaspoon fine salt

Optional for serving:

Chopped fresh chives, dill and/or parsley, and Dairy-Free Ranch Dressing and Dip (page 254)

No joke, we were once very loudly referred to as the "Crispy Potato Ladies" in a large crowd at a conference. While we both blushed wildly and, of course, laughed, we were honored to know that these fan-favorite potatoes from our blog were so life changing. What makes them so special? We think it's the savory blend of spices from our homemade ranch seasoning mix combined with the irresistibly crispy edges on the buttery potatoes, which is the perfect contrast to their smooth and creamy centers. Try the potatoes dipped in our dairy-free ranch dressing for even more ranch flavor. If you have any leftovers, toss them into your next day's breakfast, either diced alongside an omelet or topped with a fried or scrambled egg or two.

Preheat the oven to 400°F.

Place the potatoes in a 9×13-inch baking dish.

In a small bowl, stir the butter, Ranch Seasoning Mix, and ¼ teaspoon fine salt. Pour over the potatoes and toss to combine. Spread the potatoes, cut side down, in a single layer in the dish. (The fit will be snug.) Season the potatoes with a little extra salt.

Roast in the oven for 30 to 40 minutes, or until the potatoes are tender and the cut sides are golden brown. Roasting time will depend on the size of the potatoes.

Garnish the potatoes with chopped fresh chives, dill and/or parsley, and serve with Dairy-Free Ranch Dressing and Dip, if desired.

Store leftovers in an airtight container in the refrigerator for up to 3 days.

Nutrition Info: (Serving size: heaping ½ cup without the optional accompaniments) 109 calories, 4g total fat, 2g saturated fat, 174mg sodium, 17g carbs, 2g sugar, 2g fiber, 2g protein

instant pot garlic mashed potatoes

Prep Time: **10 minutes** | Cook Time: **8 minutes** | Total Time: **30 minutes, includes 10 minutes for pressure buildup** | Makes **6 servings**

GF
GrF
DFO
EF
VEG
VO
NF
NAS

2 pounds Russet or Yukon Gold potatoes, peeled and cut into 1-inch pieces

4 garlic cloves, smashed

2 cups water

Fine salt and ground black pepper

2 tablespoons unsalted butter (use vegan butter, for dairy-free and vegan)

¼ cup milk (or nondairy milk or reserved cooking water, for dairy-free and vegan)

¼ cup sour cream or plain Greek yogurt (optional; use a nondairy version or omit for dairy-free and vegan)

Tips from the Dietitians

To make the mashed potatoes on the stovetop, combine the potatoes, garlic, and ½ teaspoon salt in a large saucepan. Add enough water to cover the potatoes by 1 to 2 inches. Bring to a boil, then decrease the heat just enough to prevent the water from boiling over. Cook until the potatoes are easily pierced with a sharp knife, 15 to 20 minutes.

Make these mashed potatoes to top our Sloppy Joe Casserole (page 146) or as a base for the Slow Cooker Irish Beef Stew (page 119).

Everyone needs a solid mashed potato recipe, and this is it! These fluffy, foolproof mashed potatoes are a mainstay at Sunday suppers and holiday gatherings in our homes. They're garlicky enough to stand on their own, but not so much that they detract from your Thanksgiving turkey or any other main course. To add even more creaminess, we like to mix in a little sour cream or Greek yogurt. The advantage to using the Instant Pot is that you free up the stove and don't have to worry about the potatoes boiling over.

In a 6-quart Instant Pot, combine the potatoes, garlic, water, and ¼ teaspoon salt. Lock the lid into place and flip the vent valve to the "sealing" position. It will take about 10 minutes for the Instant Pot to build up the pressure before the timer starts counting down.

Set the Instant Pot to cook at high pressure for 8 minutes. When the timer goes off, quick-release the pressure and test the potatoes for doneness. They should be easily pierced with a knife. If the potatoes are not done, cook 1 to 2 more minutes.

Reserve ¼ cup of the cooking water, if using instead of milk. Drain the potatoes and transfer them to a medium bowl. Add the butter, milk, and sour cream, if using, and mash with a potato masher until light and fluffy. Add salt and pepper to taste.

Store leftovers in an airtight container in the refrigerator for up to 4 days or in the freezer for up to 2 months.

Nutrition Info: (Serving size: ¾ cup without the optional ingredients) 126 calories, 4g total fat, 3g saturated fat, 55mg sodium, 22g carbs, 2g sugar, 3g fiber, 3g protein

oven-roasted spaghetti squash

Prep Time: **10 minutes** | Cook Time: **40 minutes** | Total Time: **50 minutes** | Makes **4 servings**

GF
GrF
DF
EF
V
NF
NAS

1 (2- to 2½-pound) spaghetti
squash
1 tablespoon avocado oil or extra-
virgin olive oil
Fine salt

*Optional for serving as a side
dish:*
Extra-virgin olive oil, minced
garlic, and/or freshly grated or
shaved Parmesan cheese (omit
for dairy-free and vegan)

Roasting is our go-to way to prepare spaghetti squash because it comes out perfect every time: golden brown edges, with tender stands that are never watery. It's a terrific side when tossed with some really good olive oil, garlic, and freshly grated or shaved Parmesan cheese. Un-embellished, the strands form the base for our Buffalo Chicken–Stuffed Spaghetti Squash (page 81), and become a veggiecentric alternative to pasta in our Sunday Supper Beef Bolognese Sauce (page 143) and Spa-ghetti Squash Pasta and Broccoli with Dairy-Free Alfredo (page 185).

Preheat the oven to 400°F. Line a baking sheet with parchment paper and set aside.

Cut the squash in half lengthwise with a large chef's knife. Using a spoon, scoop out and discard the seeds. Brush the cut sides of the squash with the avocado oil, season with salt, and place it cut side down on the pre-pared baking sheet.

Roast in the oven for 30 to 40 minutes, or until the squash is tender and easily pierced with a fork.

Remove the squash from the oven, and once cooled enough to handle, use a fork to scrape out the strands and transfer them to a bowl. (Reserve the rinds, if making the Buffalo Chicken–Stuffed Spaghetti Squash.)

Toss the spaghetti squash with extra-virgin olive oil, minced garlic, and/or Parmesan cheese, if desired.

Store leftovers in an airtight container in the refrigerator for up to 3 days.

Nutrition Info: (Serving size: 1 cup without the optional ingredients) 49 calories, 1g total fat, 0g saturated fat, 412mg sodium, 10g carbs, 4g sugar, 2g fiber, 1g protein

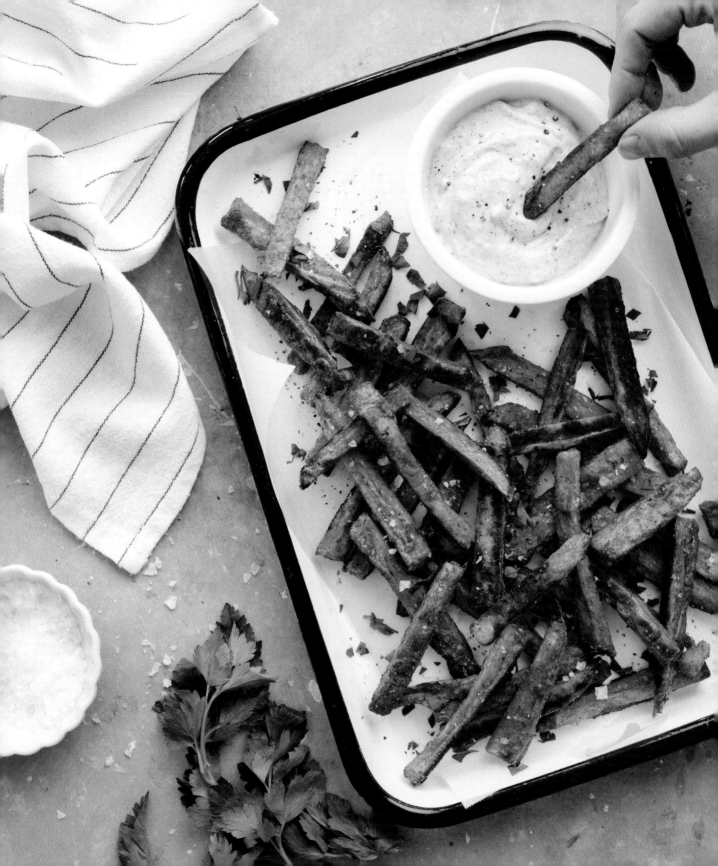

baked sweet potato fries with chipotle-lime aioli

Prep Time: **10 minutes** | Cook Time: **20 minutes** | Total Time: **30 minutes** | Makes **4 servings**

GF
GrF
DF
EFO
VEG
VO
NF
NAS

FOR THE FRIES

2 large sweet potatoes (about
   2 pounds), scrubbed clean and
   cut into ½-inch-thick sticks
2 tablespoons avocado oil or
   extra-virgin olive oil
1 tablespoon cornstarch (optional)
½ teaspoon smoked paprika
½ teaspoon garlic powder
¼ teaspoon onion powder
Fine or flaky salt

FOR THE CHIPOTLE-LIME AIOLI

⅓ cup mayonnaise (or vegan
   mayonnaise, for egg-free and
   vegan; see Tips)
½ teaspoon grated lime zest
   (½ small lime)
1 teaspoon fresh lime juice (from
   the zested lime)
1 garlic clove, grated or finely
   minced
⅛ teaspoon chipotle powder
⅛ teaspoon smoked paprika
Fine salt

Optional for serving:
Fine or flaky salt, black pepper,
   and/or chopped fresh parsley

Tips from the Dietitians
If you're looking to avoid added
sugars, use mayonnaise that is
made without sugar.

Once you start eating these, we bet you can't stop! Thick-cut sticks of sweet potato are tossed with spices and—wait for it—cornstarch, which helps these oven fries crisp up a bit more than baking them with just oil. But the best part might be the smoky chipotle-lime aioli that we serve alongside for dipping. We dare you to try and stop after just one. Serve these fries with our Simple Roast Chicken (page 93), Instant Pot Pulled Pork (page 155), or your next burger.

Make the fries: Position racks in the upper and lower thirds of the oven, and preheat it to 425°F. Line two baking sheets with parchment paper and set aside.

Place the sweet potatoes, avocado oil, cornstarch, if using, smoked paprika, garlic powder, and onion powder in a bowl. Toss well to combine. Divide the sweet potatoes between the prepared baking sheets and spread them into a single layer.

Bake on the upper and lower oven racks for 15 minutes. Flip the fries, rotate the baking sheets, and switch the positions of the baking sheets. Bake for 10 to 15 more minutes, or until the fries are brown and crispy on the edges.

Meanwhile, make the aioli: In a small bowl, combine the mayonnaise, lime zest, lime juice, garlic, chipotle powder, and smoked paprika; stir well to combine. Add fine salt to taste.

When the sweet potato fries are done, sprinkle them with fine or flaky salt, pepper, and/or chopped fresh parsley, if desired, and serve right away with the aioli.

Store leftovers in separate airtight containers in the refrigerator for up to 3 days.

Nutrition Info: (Serving size: ¼ of fries plus 1½ tablespoons aioli, without the optional ingredients) 344 calories, 18g total fat, 3g saturated fat, 806mg sodium, 41g carbs, 13g sugar, 7g fiber, 4g protein

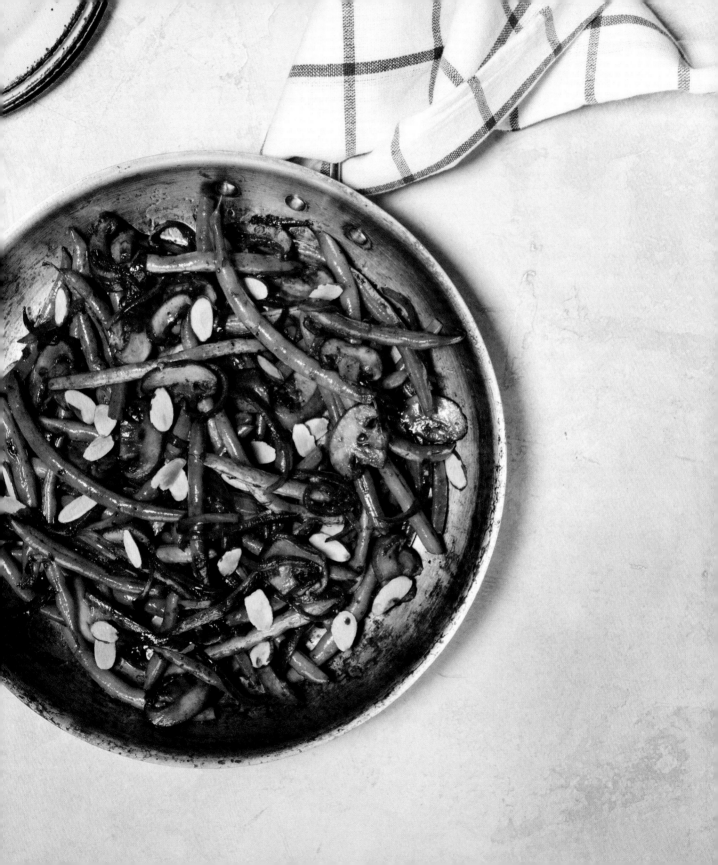

skillet green beans with balsamic & toasted almonds

Prep Time: **15 minutes** | Cook Time: **20 minutes** | Total Time: **35 minutes** | Makes **6 servings**

¼ cup sliced or slivered almonds (omit for nut-free; see Tips)

1 tablespoon avocado oil or extra-virgin olive oil

1 pound green beans, ends trimmed

¼ cup water

8 ounces cremini or button mushrooms, stems trimmed, sliced (see Tips)

½ medium red onion, sliced (1 cup)

3 garlic cloves, minced

2 tablespoons balsamic vinegar

Fine salt and ground black pepper

Tips from the Dietitians

Wipe the mushrooms clean with a damp paper towel just before using.

To make this recipe nut-free, substitute sunflower seeds for the almonds.

Like many garden growers, Stacie's brother has the tendency to grow enough green beans to feed a small army. This recipe is one of her favorite ways to make the most of that overabundance. She cooks green beans in a skillet with garlic and mushrooms, adds balsamic vinegar at the end to create a glaze, then tops the dish with toasted almonds. It's a delicious and flavorful side to spruce up a meal, like your favorite grilled meat or seafood, especially in the summer when green beans are at their peak.

Place a large skillet over medium heat. When hot, add the almonds and cook, stirring often, until they are golden and give off a toasted aroma, 6 to 8 minutes. Transfer the almonds to a plate to cool.

Wipe out the skillet and place over medium-high heat. When hot, add the avocado oil and swirl to coat the bottom. When the oil starts to shimmer, add the green beans and cook, stirring occasionally, 3 to 4 minutes. Add the water to the skillet. Bring to a simmer, then turn down the heat to medium, cover, and cook until the beans are still crisp and bright green in color, 5 to 6 minutes.

Add the mushrooms, onion, and garlic to the skillet. Increase the heat to medium-high and cook, uncovered, stirring occasionally, until the green beans are crisp-tender, 5 to 6 minutes. Add the balsamic vinegar and increase the heat slightly. Cook until the vinegar is reduced, 2 to 3 minutes. Add salt and pepper to taste.

Remove from the heat, top with the toasted almonds, and serve.

Store leftovers in an airtight container in the refrigerator for up to 3 days.

Nutrition Info: (Serving size: ¾ cup) 74 calories, 4g total fat, 0g saturated fat, 26mg sodium, 6g carbs, 4g sugar, 1g fiber, 3g protein

GF GrF DF EF V NFO NAS

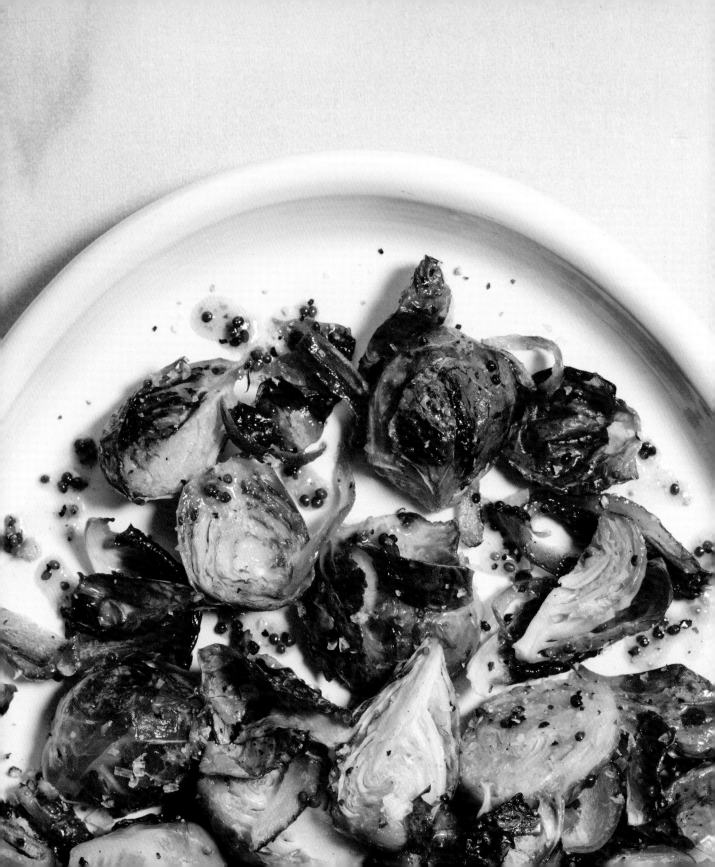

roasted brussels sprouts with maple-mustard glaze

GF
GrF
DF
EF
V
NF

Prep Time: **15 minutes** | Cook Time: **20 minutes** | Total Time: **35 minutes** | Makes **6 servings**

1½ pounds Brussels sprouts, trimmed, halved lengthwise or quartered if large (5 to 6 cups)

½ small red onion, sliced

2 garlic cloves, minced

1 tablespoon plus 1 teaspoon pure maple syrup

1 tablespoon stone-ground mustard (or Dijon mustard)

1 tablespoon avocado oil or extra-virgin olive oil

½ teaspoon fine salt, plus more as needed

¼ teaspoon ground black pepper, plus more as needed

This simple side can turn any meal from "meh" to marvelous and might just convert Brussels sprouts haters. The maple-mustard glaze takes the humble, cabbage-like vegetable to new levels. This dish is as equally suited for weeknight meals as it is for special occasions.

Preheat the oven to 400°F. Line a rimmed baking sheet with parchment paper.

Combine the Brussels sprouts, onion, and garlic on the prepared baking sheet. Set aside.

In a small bowl, combine the maple syrup, mustard, avocado oil, salt, and pepper. Whisk to combine.

Toss 2 tablespoons of the maple-mustard glaze with the vegetables. Reserve the rest for glazing after roasting.

Roast in the oven for 15 to 20 minutes, or until the Brussels sprouts are tender and slightly browned. The total time will vary depending on the size of the Brussels sprouts.

Transfer the Brussels sprouts to a serving bowl. Toss with the reserved maple-mustard glaze. Add salt and pepper to taste. Serve warm.

Store leftovers in an airtight container in the refrigerator for up to 3 days.

Nutrition Info: (Serving size: ¾ cup) 76 calories, 4g fat, 1g saturated fat, 263mg sodium, 8g carbs, 6g sugar, 1g fiber, 3g protein

crispy broccoli

Prep Time: **15 minutes** | Cook Time: **15 minutes** | Total Time: **30 minutes** | Makes **4 servings**

1 large head broccoli, trimmed
  and cut into bite-size florets the
  avocado (5 to 6 cups) or
  1 (12-ounce) bag precut
  broccoli florets, patted dry
2 garlic cloves, finely minced
1 tablespoon avocado oil or extra-
  virgin olive oil
Fine salt and ground black pepper

Roasting broccoli in the oven brings out its natural sweetness, crisps up the edges, and transforms an otherwise basic vegetable into something to look forward to. Bye-bye, boring broccoli. Hello, clean plates.

Preheat the oven to 450°F. Line a rimmed baking sheet with parchment paper.

Place the broccoli and garlic on the prepared baking sheet. Drizzle with the avocado oil and toss to coat. Spread the broccoli evenly on the baking sheet, spacing the florets apart so they do not touch each other, if possible. Season with salt and pepper.

Roast in the oven for 12 to 16 minutes, or until the broccoli stems are fork-tender and the tops are lightly browned and crispy.

Remove from the oven and serve right away.

Store leftovers in an airtight container in the refrigerator for up to 3 days.

Tips from the Dietitians
Avoid overcrowding the baking sheet to get the crispiest florets.

Nutrition Info: (Serving size: 1¼ cups) 83 calories, 3g total fat, 0g saturated fat, 56mg sodium, 12g carbs, 3g sugar, 5g fiber, 5g protein

coconut-lime rice

Prep Time: **10 minutes** | Cook Time: **20 minutes, plus 5 minutes standing time** | Total Time: **35 minutes** | Makes **4 servings**

1 cup white basmati rice
1 (14-ounce) can light coconut
  milk
¼ cup water
1 teaspoon grated lime zest
  (1 small lime)
1½ tablespoons fresh lime juice
  (from the zested lime)
½ teaspoon fine salt

Rice is nice, but it's even better when made with coconut milk and a squeeze of lime. Cooking the rice with coconut milk gives it just a hint of natural sweetness and coconut flavor to keep things interesting. We like to pair it with our Sticky Teriyaki Chicken Wings (page 209) and Quick-Pickled Carrots or Cucumbers (page 267) for a family-friendly meal.

Place the rice in a fine-mesh sieve and rinse under cool running water. Shake to remove the excess water, then transfer the rice to a medium saucepan with a lid. Add the coconut milk, water, lime zest and juice, and salt and stir to combine with the rice.

Bring the rice to a boil, cover, decrease the heat, and simmer until the rice is tender and almost all of the liquid is absorbed, 16 to 17 minutes.

Remove the saucepan from the heat and let stand, covered, for 5 minutes before removing the lid and fluffing the rice with a fork. Serve immediately.

Store leftovers in an airtight container in the refrigerator for up to 4 days.

Nutrition Info: (Serving size: ¾ cup) 213 calories, 7g total fat, 5g saturated fat, 301mg sodium, 36g carbs, 1g sugar, 1g fiber, 4g protein

GF
GrF
DF
EF
V
NF
NAS

poultry entrées

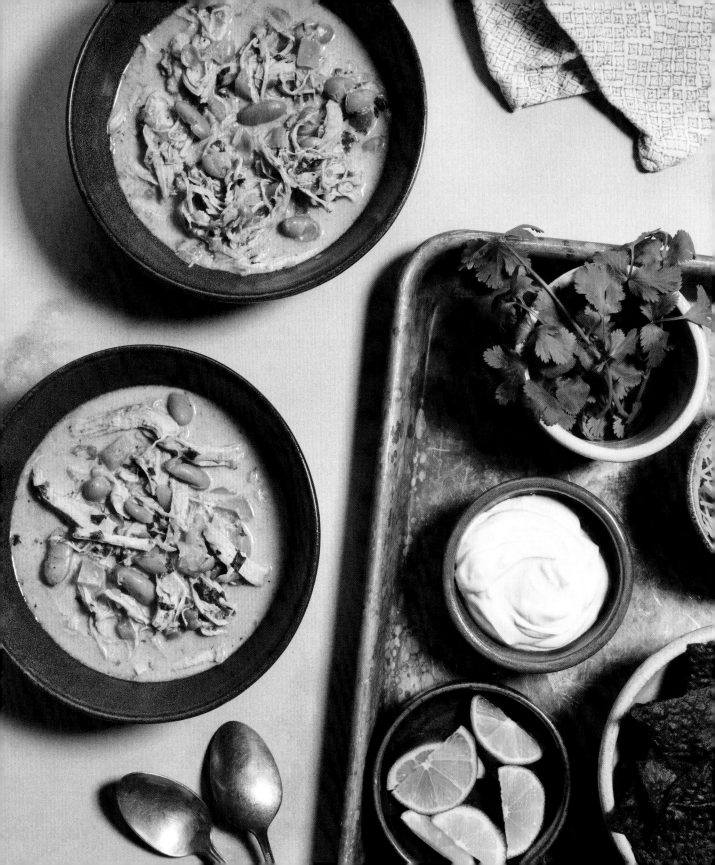

slow cooker white chicken chili with white beans

Prep Time: **15 minutes** | Cook Time: **7 hours** | Total Time: **7 hours 15 minutes** | Makes **6 servings**

1 (14-ounce) can cannellini beans, drained and rinsed

1 (4-ounce) can diced green chiles with their liquid

1 medium yellow onion, finely diced (1½ cups)

1 medium bell pepper, diced (any color; 1 cup)

6 garlic cloves, minced

1 small jalapeño, seeds and membranes removed, finely minced (see Tips)

1 tablespoon chili powder

2½ teaspoons ground cumin

1 teaspoon dried oregano

1 teaspoon fine salt, plus more as needed

½ teaspoon ground black pepper, plus more as needed

1 pound boneless, skinless chicken breasts

1½ to 2 cups low-sodium chicken broth, depending on the thickness of the chili

2 cups half-and-half (or a 14-ounce can full-fat coconut milk, for dairy-free)

1 tablespoon fresh lime juice (½ small lime)

½ cup loosely packed fresh cilantro leaves, roughly chopped

Optional toppings:
Chopped fresh cilantro leaves, lime wedges, shredded cheese (omit for dairy-free), sour cream (omit for dairy-free), and/or crushed tortilla chips (use a grain-free version or omit for grain-free)

Made with hearty beans, tender chicken, and a rich, creamy broth, this super flavorful white chili is a great alternative to the traditional beef chili with tomatoes. It's the perfect way to ward off a chill and feed a hungry family. With just fifteen minutes of prep time and the set-it-and-forget-it convenience of the slow cooker, this recipe will quickly find its way into your regular meal rotation. To make this chili dairy-free, swap out the half-and-half for a can of coconut milk—it's creamy and dreamy either way. We also give you lots of options for toppings to customize your bowl to suit your taste.

In a 6-quart slow cooker, combine the beans, green chiles and their liquid, onion, bell pepper, garlic, minced jalapeño, chili powder, cumin, oregano, salt, and black pepper. Arrange the chicken on top in a single layer.

Add 1½ cups of the broth, cover, and cook on low for 7 hours.

Transfer the chicken to a plate or bowl and shred it with two forks. Return the chicken to the slow cooker.

Add the half-and-half to the slow cooker and stir. If the chili is very thick, add the remaining ½ cup broth, cover, and cook on high for 10 to 15 minutes, or until heated through. Stir in the lime juice and cilantro. Add more salt and pepper to taste.

Serve the chili with your desired toppings. Store leftovers in an airtight container in the refrigerator for up to 4 days or in the freezer for up to 3 months.

Tips from the Dietitians
For more heat, leave the seeds and membranes in the jalapeño.

Nutrition Info: (Serving size: 1⅔ cups without the optional toppings) 285 calories, 11g total fat, 6g saturated fat, 664mg sodium, 22g carbs, 8g sugar, 4g fiber, 24g protein

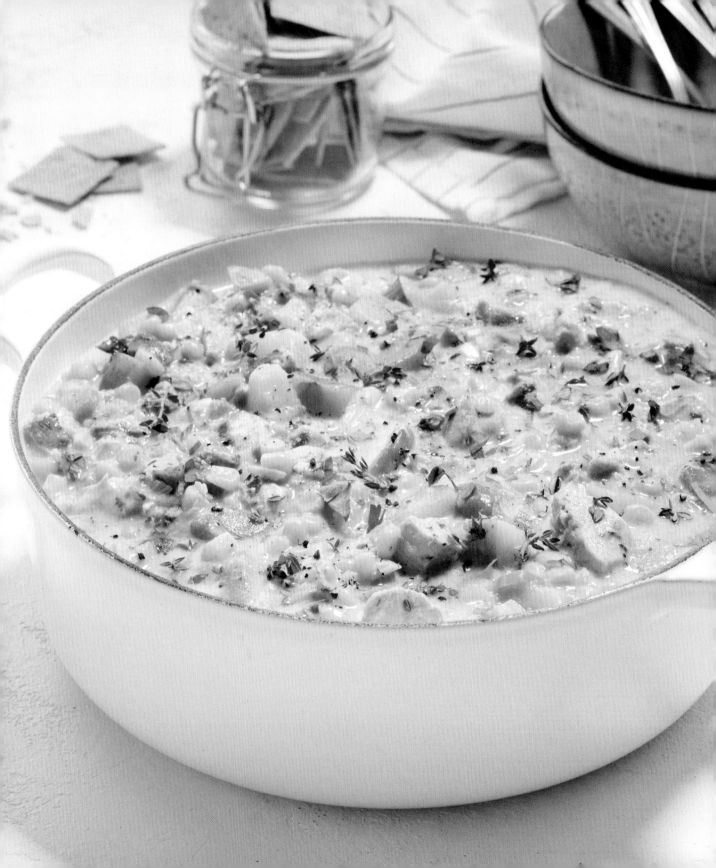

slow cooker or instant pot chicken corn chowder

Prep Time: **30 minutes** | Cook Time: **varies** | Total Time: **4 to 8 hours 30 minutes (in a slow cooker) or 45 minutes, includes 15 minutes for pressure buildup and natural release (in an Instant Pot)** | Makes **6 servings**

GF
GrF
DFO
EF
NF
NAS

1 tablespoon avocado oil or extra-virgin olive oil (if using an Instant Pot)
1 medium yellow onion, diced
2 large carrots, peeled and sliced
2 celery stalks, diced
3 garlic cloves, minced
1 pound boneless, skinless chicken breasts or thighs, cubed
1 pound red potatoes, scrubbed clean and cut into ½-inch cubes
2 cups frozen corn kernels
4 cups low-sodium chicken broth
2 tablespoons chopped fresh parsley (or 1 teaspoon dried parsley)
1 tablespoon fresh thyme leaves (or 1 teaspoon dried thyme)
½ teaspoon fine salt, plus more as needed
¼ teaspoon ground black pepper, plus more as needed
6 bacon slices (6 ounces)
1 cup heavy cream or half-and-half (or canned full-fat coconut milk, for dairy-free)

Optional for serving:
Chopped fresh parsley, fresh thyme leaves, and/or gluten-free crackers

Don't wait for the weekend to make this ultracreamy, ultracomforting chowder that combines chunks of chicken with hearty vegetables, fresh herbs, the perfect amount of corn, and crisp bacon. Simply toss all of the ingredients into the slow cooker in the morning and come home to comfort food bliss—or if you didn't plan ahead, make the Instant Pot version to put dinner on the table in under an hour.

Slow Cooker Directions

In a 6-quart slow cooker, combine the onion, carrots, celery, garlic, chicken, potatoes, and corn. Add the broth, parsley, thyme, salt, and pepper. Stir well, cover, and cook on low for 7 to 8 hours (or on high for 4 hours).

Place a medium skillet over medium-high heat. When hot, add the bacon and cook until crisp, 2 to 3 minutes per side. Remove the bacon to a paper towel–lined plate. Let cool, then crumble or roughly chop.

Stir the cream and bacon into the chowder. Add more salt and pepper to taste.

Ladle the chowder into bowls, garnish with chopped fresh parsley or fresh thyme leaves, and serve with gluten-free crackers, if desired.

Store leftovers in an airtight container in the refrigerator for up to 4 days or in the freezer for up to 3 months.

Instant Pot Directions

Select the sauté function on a 6-quart Instant Pot. When the pot is hot, add the avocado oil, onion, carrots, and celery and cook, stirring occasionally, until the onion just starts to soften, 5 to 6 minutes. Stir in the garlic and cook until fragrant, about 30 seconds. Press cancel on the Instant Pot.

Continued on the next page

Add the chicken, potatoes, corn, broth, parsley, thyme, salt, and pepper and stir well. Lock the lid in place and switch the valve to the "sealing" position.

Set the Instant Pot to cook at high pressure for 15 minutes. (It will take about 10 minutes for the Instant Pot to build up the pressure before the timer starts counting down.)

When the timer goes off, allow the pressure to naturally release for 5 minutes, then switch the vent valve to "venting" to release any residual steam.

Meanwhile, place a medium skillet over medium-high heat. When hot, add the bacon and cook until crisp, 2 to 3 minutes per side. Remove the bacon to a paper towel–lined plate. Let cool, then crumble or roughly chop.

Press cancel on the Instant Pot. Stir in the cream and bacon. Add more salt and pepper to taste.

Ladle the chowder into bowls, garnish with chopped fresh parsley or fresh thyme leaves, and serve with gluten-free crackers, if desired.

Store leftovers in an airtight container in the refrigerator for up to 4 days or in the freezer for up to 3 months.

Tips from the Dietitians

Looking for a shortcut? Use three cups of precut carrots, celery, and onions (sometimes labeled "mirepoix"), which can be found in the produce section.

If you're looking to avoid added sugars, use bacon that is made without sugar.

Nutrition Info: (Serving size: 1⅔ cups) 302 calories, 9g total fat, 4g saturated fat, 526mg sodium, 29g carbs, 8g sugar, 3g fiber, 28g protein

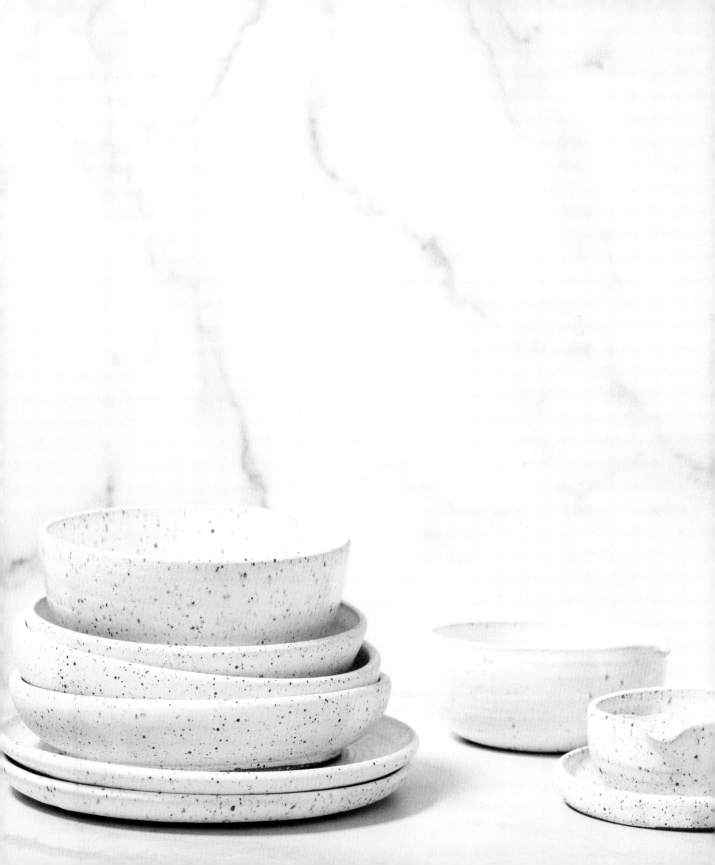

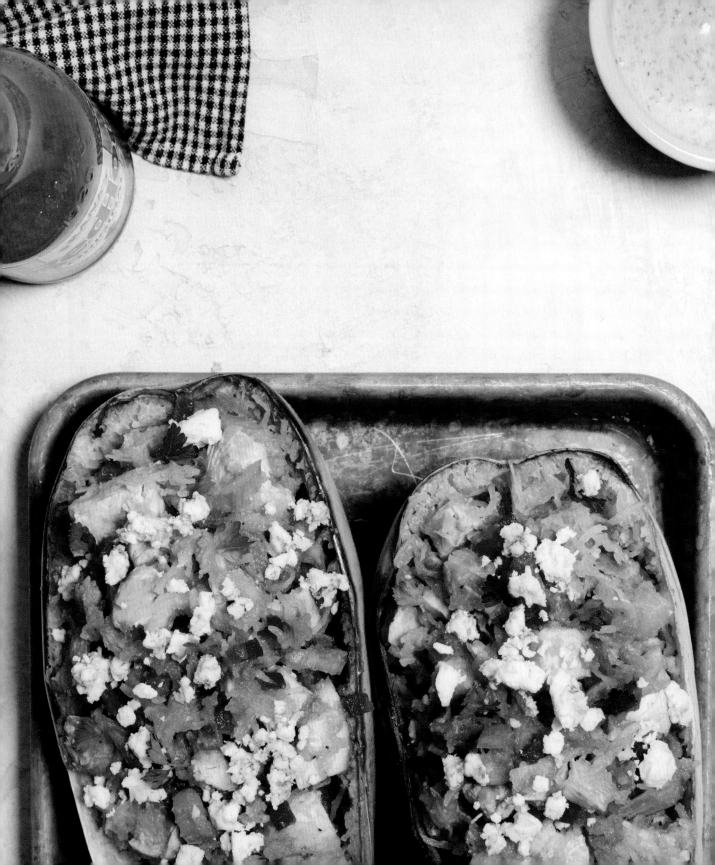

buffalo chicken–stuffed spaghetti squash

Prep Time: **20 minutes** | Cook Time: **40 minutes** | Total Time: **1 hour** | Makes **4 servings**

Oven-Roasted Spaghetti Squash
  (page 63)
1 teaspoon avocado oil or extra-
  virgin olive oil
1 pound boneless, skinless
  chicken breasts
½ cup water
½ cup cayenne pepper sauce,
  such as Frank's RedHot
2½ tablespoons unsalted butter
  (or coconut oil, for dairy-free)
1 tablespoon coconut aminos
1 teaspoon apple cider vinegar
½ teaspoon garlic powder
¼ teaspoon cayenne pepper
  (optional)
2 celery stalks, thinly sliced
  (½ cup)
2 green onions, white and green
  parts, thinly sliced
½ medium red bell pepper, finely
  diced (½ cup)

Optional toppings:
Dairy-Free Ranch Dressing and
  Dip and/or crumbled blue
  cheese (omit for dairy-free)

One of the most popular recipes on our blog, this is for the Buffalo chicken lovers who want a dish they can really tuck into and meet that Buffalo chicken craving head-on in a veggie-packed way. Drizzling the twice-baked squash with our creamy Dairy-Free Ranch Dressing and Dip (page 254) and sprinkling it with blue cheese takes it over the top. Even the most staunch spaghetti squash haters love this recipe!

After preparing the Oven-Roasted Spaghetti Squash, reserve the baking sheet, then decrease the oven temperature to 350°F. Reserve the squash rinds after scraping out the strands.

Place a medium skillet over medium-high heat. When hot, add the avocado oil and swirl to coat the bottom. Add the chicken and water and bring to a simmer. Decrease the heat enough to maintain a gentle simmer and cover the skillet. Cook until the chicken is cooked through, 15 to 18 minutes.

Transfer the chicken to a cutting board and let rest until cool enough to handle. Dice or shred into bite-size pieces, and set aside.

Meanwhile, place a small saucepan over medium heat. Add the cayenne pepper sauce, butter, coconut aminos, vinegar, garlic powder, and cayenne pepper, if using, and cook until the butter has melted. Whisk well to combine, remove from the heat, and set aside to cool.

In a large bowl, combine the Oven-Roasted Spaghetti Squash with the chicken, celery, green onions, bell pepper, and sauce. Toss well to coat, then spoon the squash mixture into the reserved squash rinds. Transfer to the reserved baking sheet and bake for 10 to 15 minutes, or until heated through.

To serve, drizzle the stuffed squash with the Dairy-Free Ranch Dressing and Dip and/or sprinkle with crumbled blue cheese, if desired.

Store leftovers in an airtight container in the refrigerator for up to 4 days.

Continued on the next page

Tips from the Dietitians
Looking for a shortcut? Swap a rotisserie chicken or leftover Simple Roast Chicken (page 93) for the chicken breasts in this recipe.

Nutrition Info: (Serving size: ¼ of the recipe without the optional toppings) 262 calories, 11g total fat, 5g saturated fat, 754mg sodium, 13g carbs, 6g sugar, 3g fiber, 26g protein

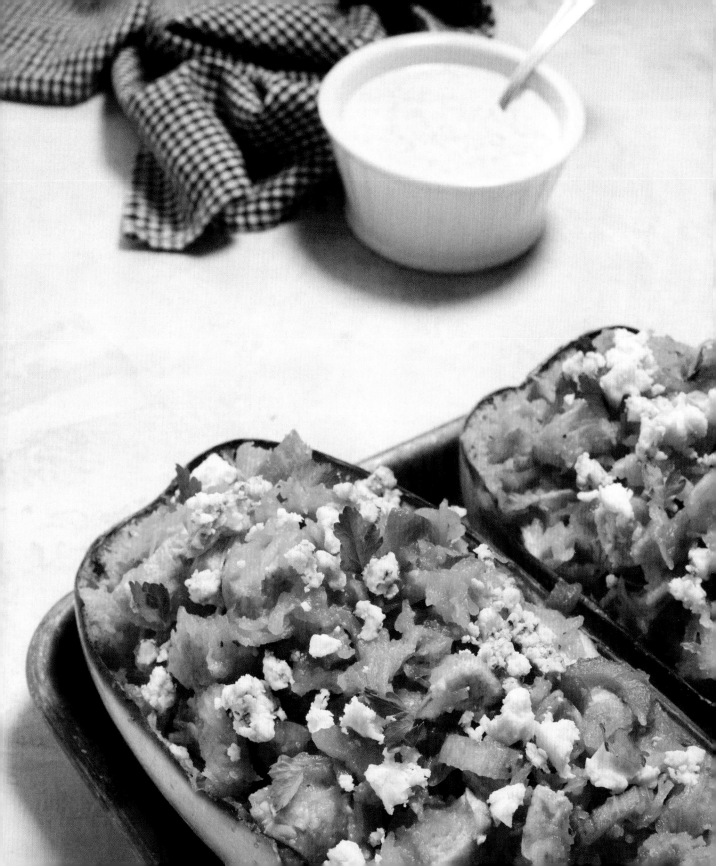

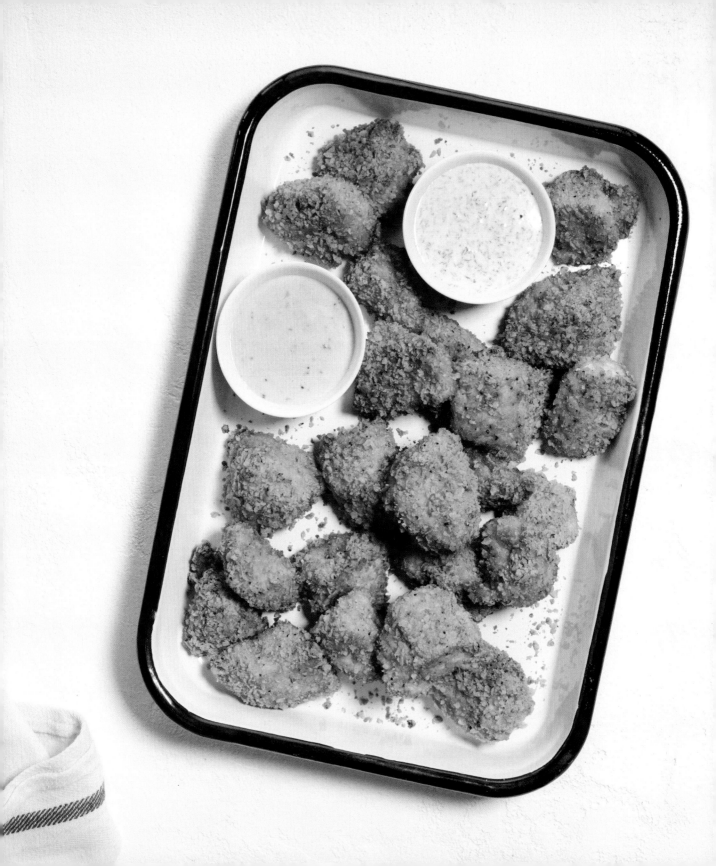

crispy baked chicken nuggets

Prep Time: **10 minutes** | Cook Time: **20 minutes** | Total Time: **30 minutes** | Makes **4 servings**

6 ounces tortilla chips (white or yellow corn; see Tips)
1½ teaspoons garlic powder
½ teaspoon onion powder
½ teaspoon fine salt
¼ teaspoon ground black pepper
¼ teaspoon paprika
1½ pounds boneless, skinless chicken breasts, cut into nugget-size pieces (about 1 inch)
2 tablespoons avocado oil or extra-virgin olive oil
Nonstick cooking spray

Optional for serving:
Honey Mustard Dressing and Dipping Sauce (page 259), Homemade Barbecue Sauce (page 260), Dairy-Free Ranch Dressing and Dip (page 254), and/or your favorite sauce, for dipping

Chicken nuggets are a family favorite, but they're not typically synonymous with a healthy meal, and they certainly aren't tailored to special diets. We're here to change that! You can make super crispy nuggets that are nonfried, gluten-free, egg-free, dairy-free, and nut-free with the help of finely crushed tortilla chips and a few key spices. You're going to love our simple cleaned-up version that is ready in under 30 minutes. Serve the nuggets with your favorite sauce or choose from our homemade dipping sauces: honey mustard, barbecue, and dairy-free ranch.

Preheat the oven to 450°F. Line a rimmed baking sheet with parchment paper and set aside.

Place the tortilla chips in a food processor and process until finely crushed. Alternatively, place the chips in a plastic zip-top bag and crush them with a rolling pin. You should have about 1½ cups.

Transfer the tortilla chip crumbs to a shallow bowl or pie plate. Add the garlic powder, onion powder, salt, pepper, and paprika and mix. Set aside.

Place the chicken in another bowl. Add the avocado oil and toss to coat.

Add a few chicken pieces at a time to the seasoned crumbs. Toss until each piece is well coated, pressing to help the crumbs adhere.

Arrange the chicken pieces on the prepared baking sheet, spacing them evenly apart. Lightly spray the top of each piece with cooking spray.

Bake for 8 minutes. Remove the baking sheet from the oven, flip over each chicken nugget, and spray the tops with cooking spray.

Bake for 8 to 10 minutes, or until the chicken is cooked through and the breading is lightly browned.

Continued on the next page

Serve the chicken nuggets with Honey Mustard Dressing and Dipping Sauce, Homemade Barbecue Sauce, Dairy-Free Ranch Dressing and Dip, or your favorite sauce, for dipping, if desired.

Store leftovers in an airtight container in the refrigerator for up to 2 days.

Tips from the Dietitians
For a grain-free option, use grain-free tortilla chips.

Nutrition Info: (Serving size: ¼ of the recipe without sauce) 448 calories, 18g total fat, 3g saturated fat, 576mg sodium, 25g carbs, 1g sugar, 2g fiber, 35g protein

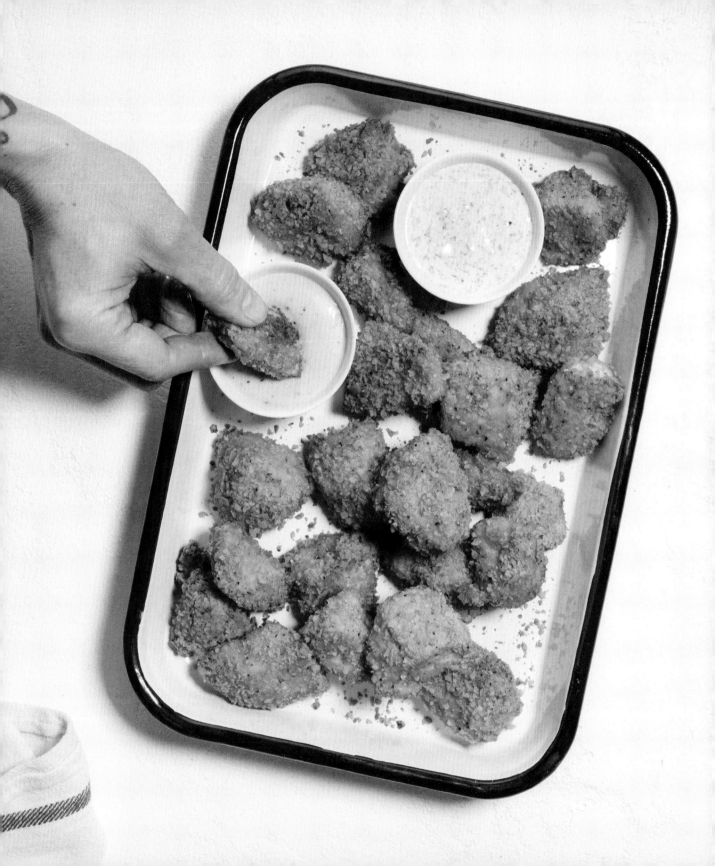

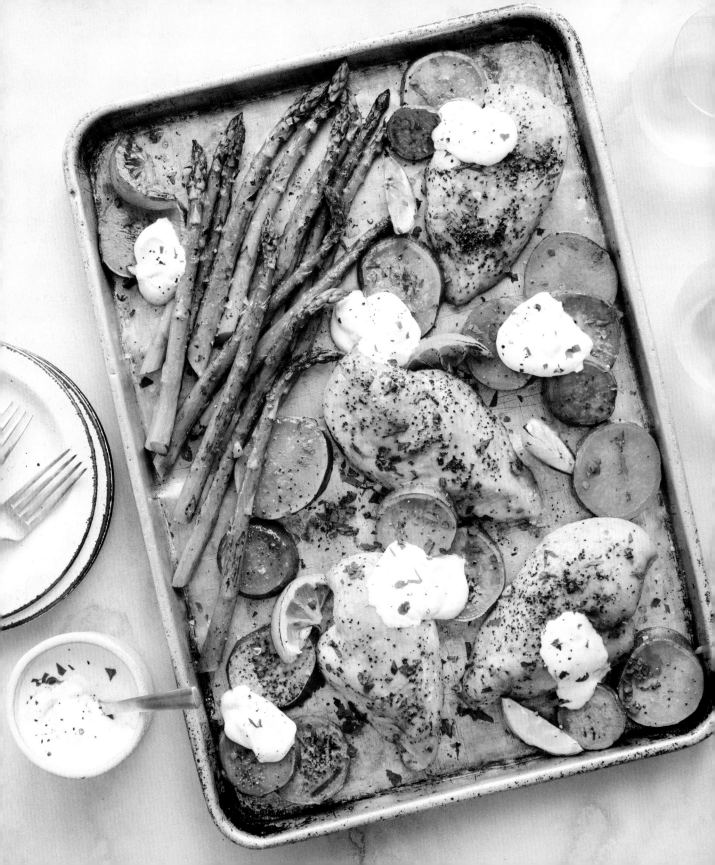

sheet pan honey-garlic chicken & vegetables with goat cheese sauce

Prep Time: **20 minutes** | Cook Time: **25 minutes** | Total Time: **45 minutes, plus 5 minutes for resting** | Makes **4 servings**

GF
GrF
DFO
EF
NF

FOR THE GOAT CHEESE SAUCE (OMIT FOR DAIRY-FREE)

2 ounces soft goat cheese, at room temperature

2 tablespoons plain yogurt

1 small garlic clove, minced or grated

1 tablespoon fresh lemon juice (¼ lemon)

1 teaspoon honey

1 teaspoon avocado oil or extra-virgin olive oil, plus more as needed

FOR THE HONEY-GARLIC MARINADE

3 tablespoons honey

2 tablespoons avocado oil or extra-virgin olive oil

2 tablespoons coconut aminos

2 tablespoons fresh lemon juice (½ lemon)

3 garlic cloves, minced

½ teaspoon fine salt

⅛ teaspoon ground black pepper

Inspired by our favorite honey-garlic marinade recipe, this meal comes together all on one sheet pan, making kitchen cleanup a breeze (you are welcome!). We nailed the timing so you'll get juicy marinated chicken breasts, tender sweet potato rounds, snappy asparagus, and lightly charred lemons for squeezing over the top. While everything bakes, make a garlicky goat cheese sauce that will have you going "mmm" after every bite. The dish is so good you'll want to hide the leftovers! This is one of Stacie's favorite recipes in the book and one she loves for weeknight dinners.

Prepare the goat cheese sauce: In a small food processor (or blender), combine the goat cheese, yogurt, garlic, lemon juice, honey, and avocado oil, and process until smooth. For a thinner consistency, add 1 more teaspoon of oil at a time and process, until your desired consistency is achieved. Set aside.

Make the marinade: In a small bowl, combine the honey, avocado oil, coconut aminos, lemon juice, garlic, salt, and pepper, and whisk to mix well. Set aside.

Prepare the chicken: If the chicken breasts vary in thickness, place them between two pieces of parchment paper and pound with the flat side of a meat tenderizer or a rolling pin until even in thickness.

Place the chicken in a shallow dish and add ¼ cup of the marinade (reserve the rest for the vegetables). Toss to coat and let marinate in the refrigerator for 30 minutes while you prepare the remaining ingredients.

Preheat the oven to 425°F. Line a rimmed baking sheet with parchment paper.

Continued on the next page

FOR THE CHICKEN AND VEGETABLES

1¼ pounds boneless, skinless chicken breasts (3 to 4 breasts)

2 medium sweet potatoes (10 to 12 ounces each), scrubbed clean and sliced into rounds about ½ inch thick

1 medium lemon, quartered

1 pound asparagus, ends trimmed

Fine salt and ground black pepper

Chopped fresh parsley, for serving

After the marinating time is up, arrange the chicken in a single layer on one side of the prepared baking sheet. Discard the marinade.

Prepare the vegetables: In a medium bowl, combine the sweet potatoes with 2 tablespoons of the reserved marinade, and toss to coat. Arrange the potatoes in a single layer on the other side of the baking sheet. Add the lemon wedges to the baking sheet. Season the sweet potatoes and chicken with salt and pepper.

Roast in the oven for 12 minutes.

Remove the baking sheet from the oven. Flip the sweet potatoes and add the asparagus wherever it fits on the baking sheet. Lightly brush the asparagus, sweet potatoes, and chicken with a little more of the marinade, reserving some for broiling. Roast for 10 to 15 minutes, or until an instant-read thermometer inserted into the center of the largest breast registers 165°F.

Remove the baking sheet from the oven and switch the oven to broil. Brush the chicken with the remaining marinade. Broil for 2 minutes, watching closely so nothing on the baking sheet burns.

Allow the chicken to rest for 5 minutes, then serve with the sweet potatoes, asparagus, and lemon wedges. Top the chicken and/or vegetables with the goat cheese sauce and garnish with the parsley.

Store leftover chicken and vegetables in an airtight container in the refrigerator for up to 3 days. Store any leftover sauce in an airtight container in the refrigerator for up to 5 days.

Nutrition Info: (Serving size: ¼ of the recipe plus 2 tablespoons sauce) 378 calories, 11g total fat, 4g saturated fat, 775mg sodium, 36g carbs, 8g sugar, 6g fiber, 33g protein

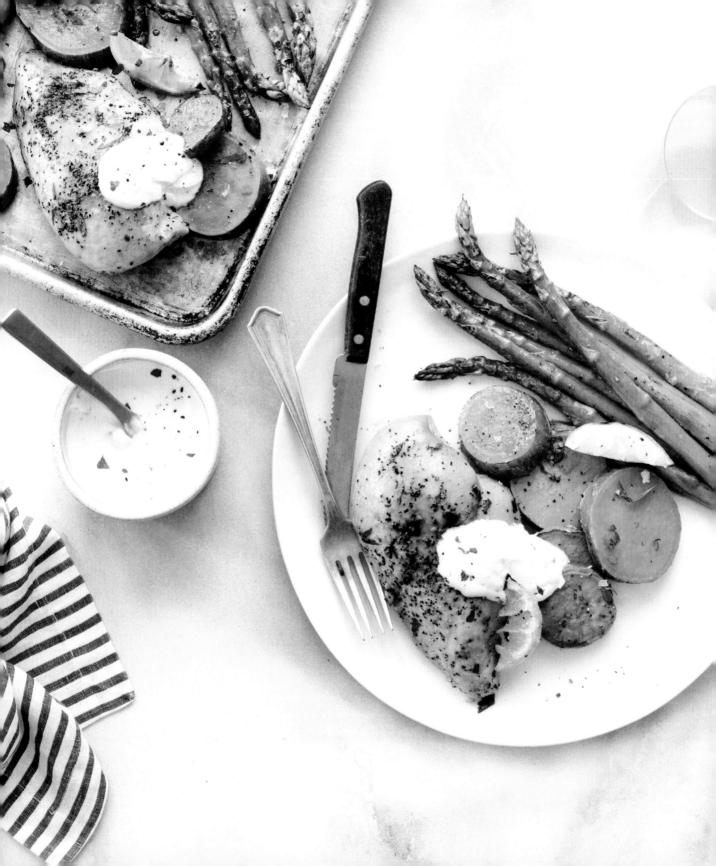

homestyle chicken & rice soup

Prep Time: **15 minutes** | Cook Time: **25 minutes** | Total Time: **40 minutes** | Makes **6 servings**

2 pounds bone-in chicken thighs, skin removed

8 cups low-sodium chicken broth

4 medium carrots, peeled and thinly sliced (1½ cups)

1 medium onion, diced (1½ cups)

3 celery stalks, diced (¾ cup)

⅔ cup long-grain white rice (or white basmati rice)

4 garlic cloves, minced

1½ teaspoons dried parsley

¾ teaspoon dried thyme

½ teaspoon salt, plus more as needed

¼ teaspoon ground black pepper, plus more as needed

Basic but not boring, a big bowl of comforting chicken soup always hits the spot, especially when it's a snow day or you or someone you love is under the weather. This one-pot wonder made with tender chunks of chicken swimming in a sea of vegetables and rice will be a welcome addition to your rotation of simple weeknight meals. Leftovers, when put in a thermos, make a packed lunch something to look forward to.

Combine the chicken, broth, carrots, onion, celery, rice, garlic, parsley, thyme, salt, and pepper in a large pot. Cover and bring just to a boil over high heat.

Decrease the heat just enough to maintain a gentle simmer and cook until the rice and vegetables are tender, 20 to 25 minutes. As the soup simmers, use a large spoon to skim off any foam that collects on the surface.

Remove the soup from the heat. Using tongs or a slotted spoon, transfer the chicken to a plate or shallow bowl. Allow the chicken to rest until cool enough to handle, then remove the meat from the bones and cut it into ½-inch pieces. Discard the bones.

Return the chicken to the soup. Add salt and pepper to taste, and serve.

Store leftovers in an airtight container in the refrigerator for up to 4 days or in the freezer for up to 3 months.

Nutrition Info: (Serving size: 1¾ cups) 232 calories, 7g total fat, 2g saturated fat, 573mg sodium, 19g carbs, 3g sugar, 1g fiber, 23g protein

simple roast chicken

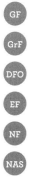

Prep Time: **15 minutes** | Cook Time: **55 minutes** | Total Time: **1 hour 10 minutes, plus 10 minutes for resting** | Makes **6 servings**

1 (4- to 4½-pound) whole chicken, giblets removed

Avocado oil or extra-virgin olive oil

Fine salt and ground black pepper

1 tablespoon unsalted butter (omit for dairy-free)

2 teaspoons fresh thyme leaves or chopped fresh rosemary leaves (optional)

Jessica had a green coffee mug in college with a Leonardo da Vinci quote: "Simplicity is the ultimate sophistication." While that mug disappeared some time ago during her travels, that quote has stuck with her ever since. This simple roast chicken embodies that saying. Just a little oil, butter, salt, and pepper is all you need. The hot oven creates deep golden skin that's crisp and crackling, which when pulled away reveals flavorful, tender meat. This recipe is her go-to for Sunday dinners with family. Just one taste and you'll see why!

Preheat the oven to 450°F.

Pat the chicken dry inside and out with paper towels. Place the chicken, breast side up, in a roasting pan or large cast-iron skillet. Rub the chicken all over with avocado oil, then season with salt and pepper.

Roast, uncovered and undisturbed, for 45 to 55 minutes, or until an instant-read thermometer inserted into the thickest part of the breast registers 165°F.

Remove the chicken from the oven and add the butter and thyme, if using, to the pan juices. Allow the butter to melt, then spoon the pan juices over the chicken to baste it.

Allow the chicken to rest for 10 minutes before serving.

Store leftovers in an airtight container in the refrigerator for up to 4 days.

Tips from the Dietitians
Got leftover chicken? Use it to make Curried Chicken Salad (page 99), Strawberry Poppy Seed Chicken Salad (page 95), or Buffalo Chicken–Stuffed Spaghetti Squash (page 81).

Nutrition Info: (Serving size: 5 ounces mixed white and dark meat chicken) 262 calories, 14g total fat, 4g saturated fat, 750mg sodium, 1g carbs, 0g sugar, 0g fiber, 29g protein

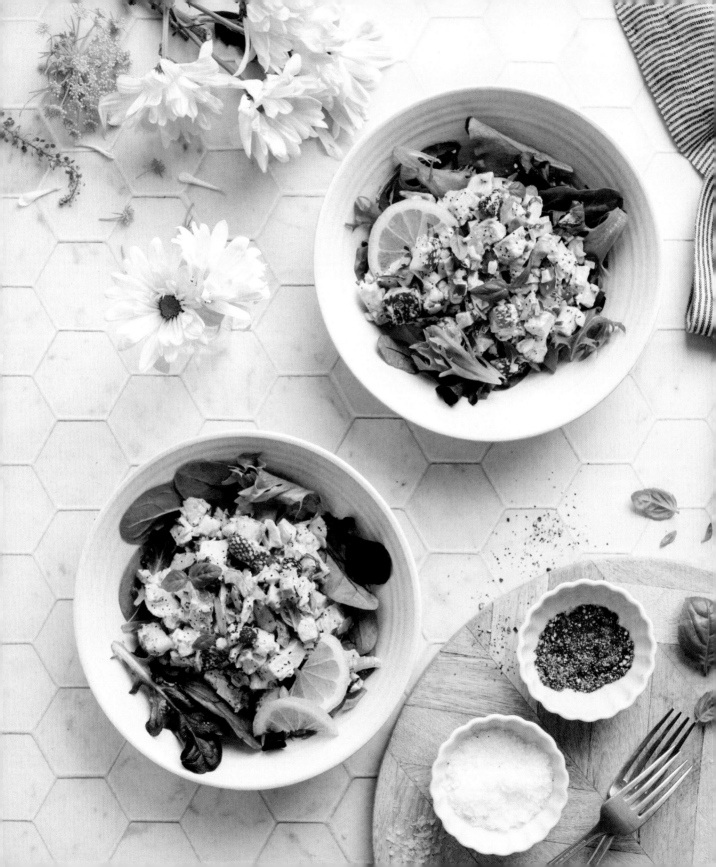

strawberry poppy seed chicken salad

Prep Time: **15 minutes** | Cook Time: **20 minutes** | Total Time: **35 minutes** | Makes **4 servings**

GF
GrF
DF
EFO
NFO
NAS

FOR THE CHICKEN

12 ounces boneless, skinless chicken breast

Fine salt and ground black pepper

1 tablespoon avocado oil or extra-virgin olive oil

½ cup low-sodium chicken broth or water

¼ cup sliced or slivered almonds (omit for nut-free; see Tips)

½ cup diced strawberries

¼ cup finely diced celery

2 tablespoons finely diced red onion

2 tablespoons chopped basil leaves

FOR THE DRESSING

⅓ cup mayonnaise (or vegan mayonnaise, for egg-free; see Tips)

2 tablespoons fresh lemon juice (½ medium lemon)

1 teaspoon poppy seeds

Optional for serving:

Butter lettuce or green leaf lettuce leaves, and/or gluten-free or grain-free tortillas, sandwich bread, or crackers

We revamp ordinary chicken salad with sweet strawberries, fresh basil, toasted almonds, and a creamy poppy seed dressing that has a lemony zing. This chicken salad is super quick to make if you start with cooked chicken. We like to serve it tucked into a crisp lettuce leaf for a light yet satisfying meal.

Prepare the chicken: Pat the chicken dry with a paper towel. If the chicken breasts vary in thickness, place them between two pieces of parchment paper and pound with the flat side of a meat tenderizer or a rolling pin until even in thickness. Season both sides of the chicken with salt and pepper.

Place a medium skillet over medium-high heat. When hot, add the avocado oil and swirl to coat the bottom. When the oil starts to shimmer, add the chicken breasts. Decrease the heat slightly and cook, undisturbed, until the chicken easily releases from the pan, 4 to 5 minutes. Flip and cook, undisturbed, until lightly browned on the second side, 3 to 4 minutes.

Add the broth to the skillet and bring to a simmer, then cover the skillet and decrease the heat to medium-low to maintain a simmer. Cook, covered, until the chicken is no longer pink inside and an instant-read thermometer registers 165°F when inserted in the center of the largest breast, 8 to 10 minutes.

Transfer the chicken to a cutting board and let rest until cool enough to handle, about 10 minutes. Dice the chicken and refrigerate in a bowl until completely cool. Meanwhile, prepare the remaining ingredients.

Place a small skillet over medium heat. When hot, add the almonds and cook, stirring often, until they are golden and give off a toasted aroma, 6 to 8 minutes. Transfer the almonds to a plate to cool.

Continued on the next page

In a medium bowl, combine the chicken, almonds, strawberries, celery, onion, and basil. Set aside.

Make the dressing: In a small bowl, combine the mayonnaise, lemon juice, and poppy seeds and stir to mix well.

Pour the dressing over the chicken mixture and toss gently until well combined. Add salt and pepper to taste.

Serve the chicken salad tucked in butter lettuce or green leaf lettuce leaves or tortillas, between sandwich bread, or on top of crackers, if desired.

Store leftovers in an airtight container in the refrigerator for up to 3 days.

Tips from the Dietitians

For a creamier chicken salad, add 1 to 2 more tablespoons of mayonnaise to the dressing. If you're looking to avoid added sugars, use mayonnaise that is made without sugar.

For a shortcut, use 2 cups of cooled, diced leftover chicken or rotisserie chicken.

To make this recipe nut-free, substitute sunflower seeds for the almonds.

Nutrition Info: (Serving size: ¾ cup without the optional accompaniments) 254 calories, 17g total fat, 2g saturated fat, 151mg sodium, 3g carbs, 1g sugar, 1g fiber, 21g protein

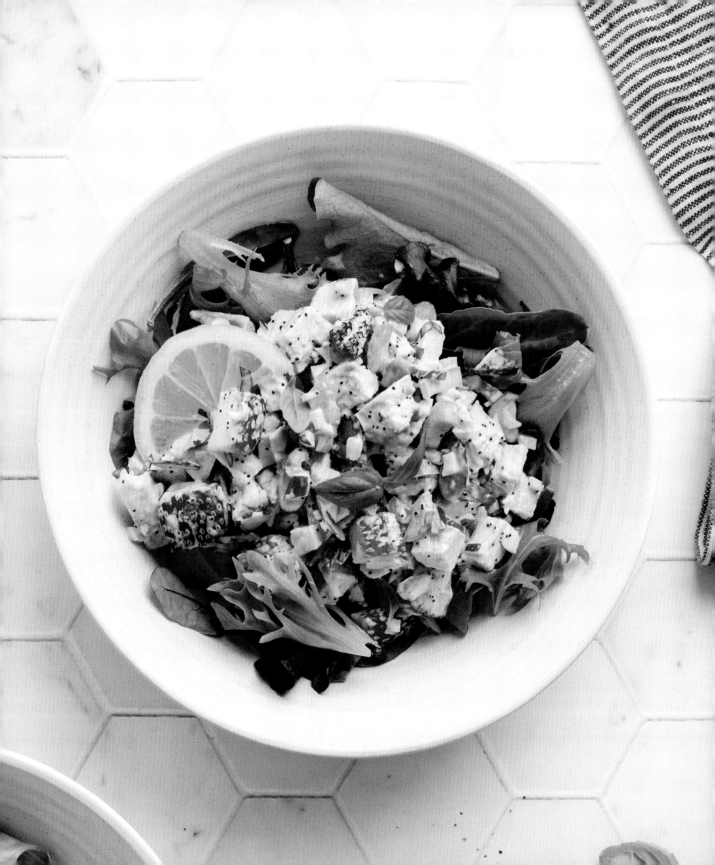

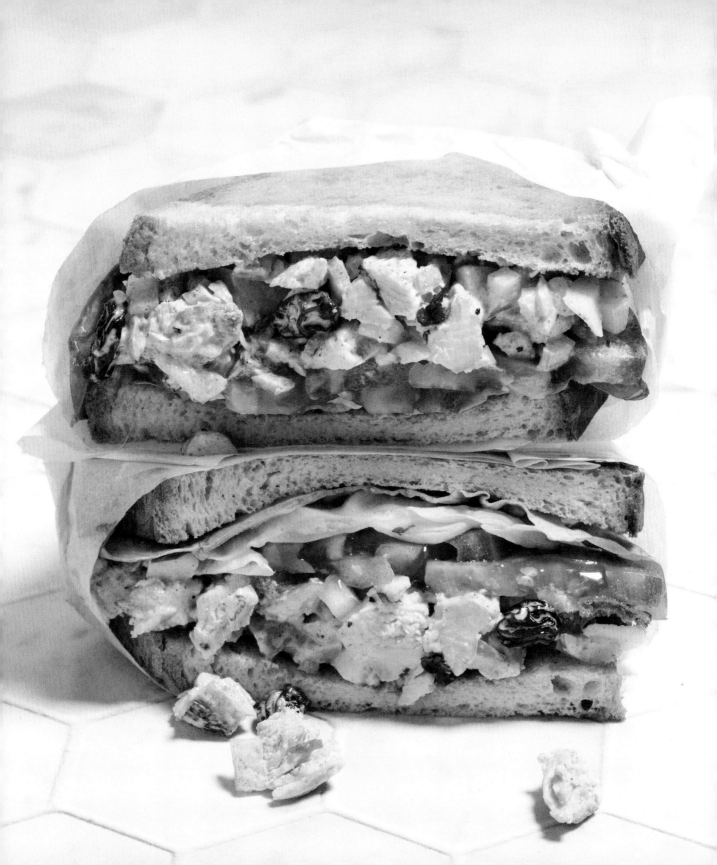

curried chicken salad

Prep Time: **15 minutes** | Cook Time: **20 minutes** | Total Time: **35 minutes** | Makes **4 servings**

GF
GrF
DF
EFO
NFO
NAS

FOR THE CHICKEN
12 ounces boneless, skinless chicken breast
Fine salt and ground black pepper
1 tablespoon avocado oil or extra-virgin olive oil
½ cup low-sodium chicken broth or water
¾ cup diced apple, any kind (½ medium apple)
¼ cup finely diced celery
¼ cup roasted cashews, chopped (omit for nut-free; see Tips)
3 tablespoons dark raisins
2 tablespoons finely diced red onion
2 tablespoons chopped fresh cilantro leaves

FOR THE DRESSING
⅓ cup mayonnaise (or vegan mayonnaise, for egg-free; see Tips)
2 tablespoons fresh lime juice (1 medium lime)
1½ teaspoons curry powder
Fine salt and ground black pepper

Optional for serving:
Butter lettuce or green leaf lettuce leaves and/or gluten-free or grain-free tortillas, sandwich bread, or crackers

With Indian-inspired flavors, this unique chicken salad is both delicious and nutritious made with antioxidant-rich curry powder, crisp vegetables, and crunchy cashew. The combination of apples and raisins creates that sweet and savory flavor that will keep you coming back to this recipe. Enjoy the chicken salad as a sandwich with gluten-free bread, in lettuce wraps, or with your favorite crackers.

Prepare the chicken: Pat the chicken dry with a paper towel. If the chicken breasts vary in thickness, place them between two pieces of parchment paper and pound with the flat side of a meat tenderizer or a rolling pin until even in thickness. Season both sides of the chicken with salt and pepper.

Place a medium skillet over medium-high heat. When hot, add the avocado oil and swirl to coat the bottom. When the oil starts to shimmer, add the chicken breasts. Decrease the heat slightly and cook, undisturbed, until the chicken easily releases from the pan, 4 to 5 minutes. Flip and cook, undisturbed, until lightly browned on the second side, 3 to 4 minutes.

Add the broth to the skillet and bring to a simmer, then cover the skillet and decrease the heat to medium-low to maintain a simmer. Cook, covered, until the chicken is no longer pink inside and an instant-read thermometer registers 165°F when inserted in the center of the largest breast, 8 to 10 minutes.

Transfer the chicken to a cutting board and let rest until cool enough to handle, about 10 minutes.

Dice the chicken and refrigerate in a bowl until completely cool. While the chicken is chilling, prepare the remaining ingredients.

In a medium bowl, combine the apple, celery, cashews, raisins, onion, and cilantro. When the chicken is chilled, add to the bowl and combine. Set aside.

Continued on the next page

Make the dressing: In a small bowl, combine the mayonnaise, lime juice, and curry powder and stir to mix well.

Pour the dressing over the chicken mixture. Toss gently until well combined. Add salt and pepper to taste.

Serve the chicken salad tucked in butter lettuce or green leaf lettuce leaves or tortillas, between sandwich bread, or on top of crackers, if desired.

Store leftovers in an airtight container in the refrigerator for up to 3 days.

Tips from the Dietitians

For a creamier chicken salad, add 1 to 2 more tablespoons mayonnaise to the dressing. If you're looking to avoid added sugars, use mayonnaise that is made without sugar.

For a shortcut, use 2 cups of cooled, diced leftover chicken or rotisserie chicken.

To make this nut-free, substitute sunflower seeds for the cashews.

Nutrition Info: (Serving size: heaping ¾ cup without the optional accompaniments) 378 calories, 27g total fat, 4g saturated fat, 222mg sodium, 12g carbs, 7g sugar, 1g fiber, 21g protein

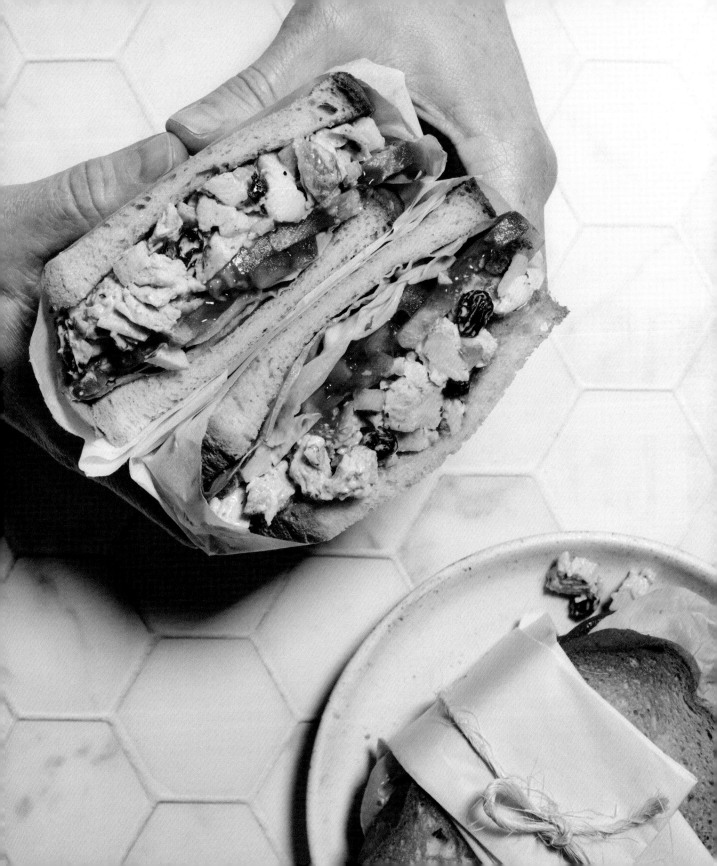

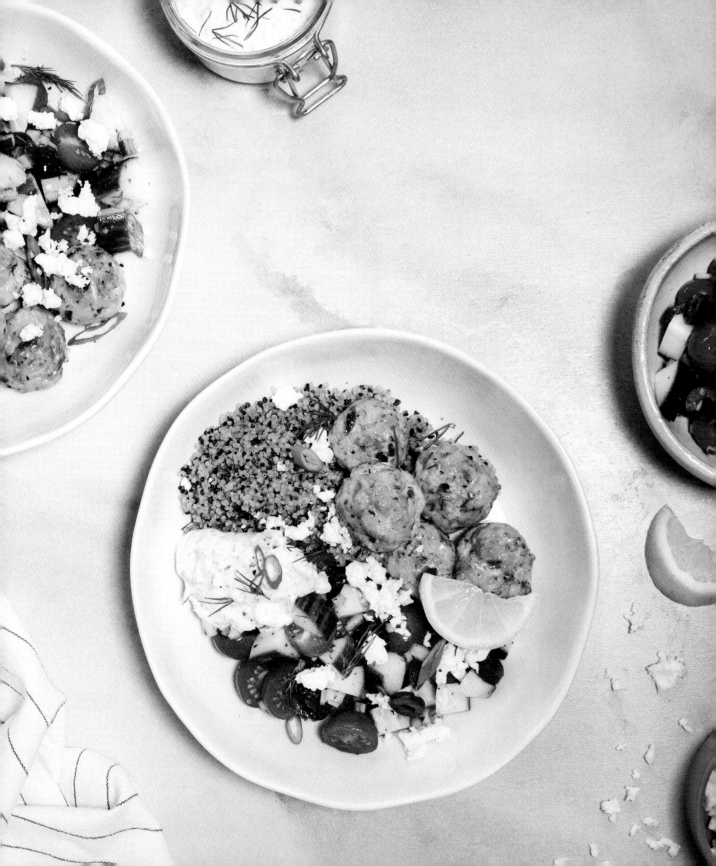

greek chicken meatball bowls with tzatziki

Prep Time: **30 minutes** | Cook Time: **15 minutes** | Total Time: **45 minutes** | Makes **4 servings**

GF
DFO
EF
NF
NAS

FOR THE TZATZIKI
1 cup grated English cucumber, squeezed to remove the excess liquid
1 cup plain Greek yogurt (use nondairy yogurt for dairy-free)
1 tablespoon extra-virgin olive oil
3 tablespoons fresh lemon juice
1 teaspoon dried dill
1 garlic clove, finely minced
¼ teaspoon fine salt
⅛ teaspoon ground black pepper

FOR THE CHICKEN MEATBALLS
1 pound ground chicken
2 green onions, thinly sliced
2 garlic cloves, minced
1 teaspoon dried oregano
¼ teaspoon fine salt
⅛ teaspoon ground black pepper
Pinch of crushed red pepper flakes (optional)

FOR THE QUINOA AND GREEK SALAD
¾ cup quinoa
2 cups diced English cucumber
2 cups grape tomatoes, halved
¼ cup finely minced red onion
⅓ cup pitted sliced kalamata olives
¼ cup Greek Vinaigrette and Marinade (page 258)

Optional, for serving:
½ cup crumbled feta cheese (omit for dairy-free), lemon wedges, sliced green onions, and/or fresh dill

We've channeled the flavors of the mall food court gyros that we loved as teens into these vibrant bowls. We replaced the usual shaved pork or chicken with flavorful chicken meatballs and ditched the pita for fluffy quinoa. We round out the bowls with fresh vegetables, salty-briny olives, feta cheese, and creamy tzatziki for a winning combo.

Preheat the oven to 350°F. Line a rimmed baking sheet with parchment paper. (While the oven is heating, this is a good time to prepare the Greek Vinaigrette and Marinade, for the quinoa.)

Make the tzatziki: Combine the cucumber, yogurt, oil, lemon juice, dill, garlic, salt, and pepper in a small bowl and stir well. Refrigerate until ready to serve.

Make the meatballs: In a medium bowl, combine the chicken, green onions, garlic, oregano, salt, black pepper, and red pepper flakes, if using, and mix to combine.

Shape the chicken mixture into 16 balls (about 1 ounce each) and place on the prepared baking sheet. Bake for 13 to 15 minutes, or until the meatballs are no longer pink in the center.

Meanwhile, make the quinoa: Prepare the quinoa according to the package directions.

While the quinoa is cooking, make the Greek salad: In another medium bowl, combine the cucumbers, tomatoes, red onion, and olives with the Greek Vinaigrette and toss to coat.

Divide the meatballs, quinoa, and salad among four bowls. Top each with ¼ cup of the tzatziki and sprinkle with 2 tablespoons of the feta, if using, and any other optional toppings.

Store leftovers in separate airtight containers in the refrigerator for up to 3 days.

Nutrition Info: (Serving size: ¼ of the recipe) 525 calories, 28g total fat, 7g saturated fat, 716mg sodium, 34g carbs, 8g sugar, 3g fiber, 33g protein

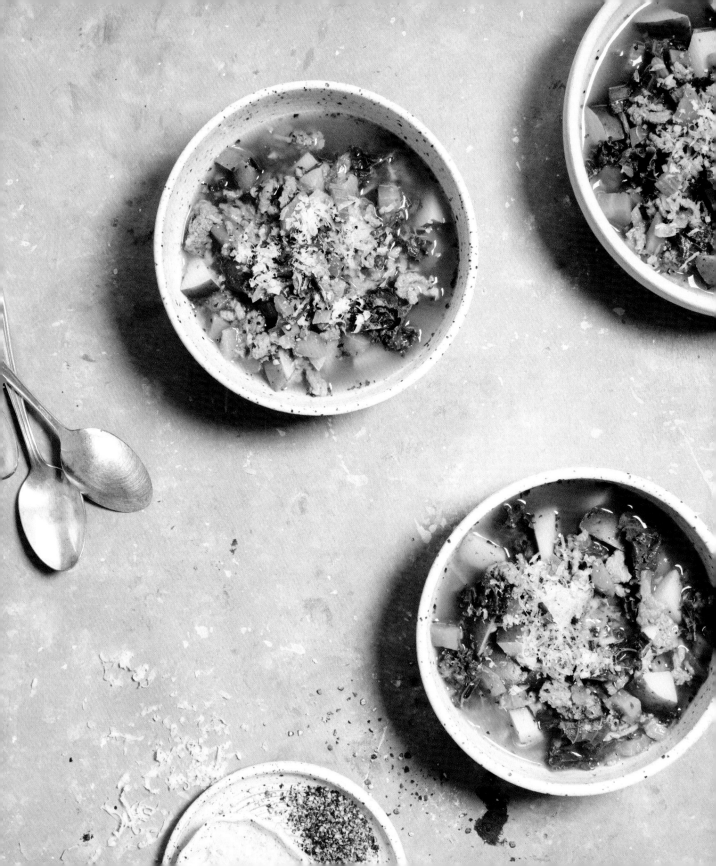

italian turkey sausage & vegetable soup

Prep Time: **20 minutes** | Cook Time: **40 minutes** | Total Time: **60 minutes** | Makes **4 servings**

GF GrF DFO EF NF NAS

FOR THE HOMEMADE TURKEY SAUSAGE

2 teaspoons avocado oil or extra-virgin olive oil

1 pound ground turkey (we use 93% lean/7% fat)

1½ teaspoons dried Italian seasoning

1 teaspoon garlic powder

¾ teaspoon dried fennel seeds, lightly crushed

1 teaspoon fine salt

¼ teaspoon ground black pepper

¼ teaspoon crushed red pepper flakes

FOR THE SOUP

1 tablespoon avocado oil or extra-virgin olive oil

½ medium yellow onion, diced

3 medium carrots, peeled and diced (1½ cups)

2 celery stalks, diced

4 garlic cloves, minced

12 ounces red or Yukon Gold potatoes, scrubbed clean and cut into ½-inch cubes (2½ cups)

1 teaspoon dried Italian seasoning

½ teaspoon fine salt

4 cups low-sodium chicken broth

1 small bunch curly kale, ribs removed and leaves chopped (3 cups)

Optional for serving:
Freshly grated Parmesan cheese (omit for dairy-free)

This satisfying soup features hearty fall and winter vegetables and homemade Italian turkey sausage. Making your own sausage means you can control the ingredients and steer clear of preservatives, fillers, and added sugars. After a day of skiing, Jessica and her family love to warm up with big bowls of this soup topped with Parmesan cheese. Thankfully, it's quick to make and uses long-storing vegetables she already has on hand because her daughters request it often.

Make the homemade turkey sausage: Place a large pot over medium-high heat. When hot, add the avocado oil and swirl to coat the bottom.

Add the turkey, Italian seasoning, garlic powder, fennel seeds, salt, black pepper, and crushed red pepper flakes. Using a wooden spoon, break up the turkey and mix the spices into it. Cook, stirring occasionally, until the meat is no longer pink, 8 to 9 minutes. Transfer the sausage to a plate and set aside.

Make the soup: Wipe the pot clean with a paper towel then return it to medium-high heat. When hot, add the avocado oil and swirl to coat the bottom. Add the onion, carrots, celery, and garlic and cook, stirring occasionally, until the onion starts to soften, about 7 minutes.

Add the sausage, potatoes, Italian seasoning, salt, and broth to the pot. Increase the heat to high and bring just to a boil. Decrease the heat, partially cover the pot, and simmer until the vegetables are tender, 17 to 20 minutes.

Remove the pot from the heat and stir in the kale. Let the soup stand until the kale wilts, 3 to 4 minutes.

Serve the soup with Parmesan cheese, if desired.

Store leftovers in an airtight container in the refrigerator for up to 4 days or in the freezer for up to 3 months.

Nutrition Info: (Serving size: 2 cups without the optional cheese) 314 calories, 13g total fat, 3g saturated fat, 535mg sodium, 18g carbs, 4g sugar, 2g fiber, 30g protein

fire-roasted turkey & bean chili

Prep Time: **20 minutes** | Cook Time: **20 minutes** | Total Time: **40 minutes** | Makes **6 servings**

GF
GrF
DF
EF
NF
NAS

2 teaspoons avocado oil or extra-virgin olive oil

1 pound ground turkey (we use 93% lean/7% fat)

1 medium bell pepper, diced (any color; 1½ cups)

½ medium red onion, diced (1 cup)

1 small zucchini, diced (1 cup)

1 small yellow squash, diced (1 cup)

3 garlic cloves, minced

2 cups low-sodium chicken or beef broth

1 (15-ounce) can fire-roasted diced tomatoes with their juices

1 (15-ounce) can tomato sauce

1 (15-ounce) can black beans, drained and rinsed

1 (15-ounce) can pinto beans, drained and rinsed

3 tablespoons chili powder

1 tablespoon ground cumin

1 teaspoon dried oregano

¼ teaspoon ground black pepper

1 teaspoon fine salt, plus more as needed

Dash of your favorite hot sauce or a pinch or two of cayenne pepper (optional)

Optional toppings
Chopped fresh cilantro leaves, sliced or diced avocado, pickled or fresh jalapeño slices, sour cream (omit for dairy-free), shredded cheese (omit for dairy-free), crushed tortilla chips (use a grain-free version or omit for grain-free), and/or lime wedges

Our hopped-up version of chili features lean ground turkey for plenty of protein, and loads of vegetables for vitamins, minerals, and fiber. While it may be healthier than your average bowl of chili, it definitely doesn't taste like health food thanks to its thick, rich tomato base and warm chili spices. Jessica loves to make a batch to take camping for an easy, family friendly meal that can be reheated on the camp stove after a long day of exploring.

Place a large saucepan or Dutch oven over medium-high heat. When hot, add the avocado oil and swirl to coat the bottom. Add the turkey, break it up with a wooden spoon, then add the bell pepper, onion, zucchini, yellow squash, and garlic. Cook, stirring occasionally, until the onion is translucent and the turkey is no longer pink, 7 to 8 minutes.

Add the broth, diced tomatoes with their juices, the tomato sauce, black beans, pinto beans, chili powder, cumin, oregano, black pepper, and salt and stir to combine. Bring the mixture to a gentle simmer, adjusting the heat as necessary. Cover and cook until the zucchini and yellow squash are tender, about 12 minutes. Add more salt to taste. Add the hot sauce or cayenne pepper, if desired, for a spicier chili.

Serve with your desired toppings.

Store leftovers in an airtight container in the refrigerator for up to 4 days or in the freezer for up to 3 months.

Nutrition Info: (Serving size: ¾ cups without the optional toppings) 325 calories, 9g total fat, 2g saturated fat, 437mg sodium, 34g carbs, 8g sugar, 11g fiber, 25g protein

easy egg roll bowls

Prep Time: **10 minutes** | Cook Time: **20 minutes** | Total Time: **30 minutes** | Makes **4 servings**

GF
GrF
DF
EF
NF
NAS

½ cup coconut aminos

2 tablespoons toasted sesame oil

2 tablespoons rice vinegar

5 garlic cloves, minced

1 tablespoon grated peeled fresh ginger (or 1 teaspoon ground ginger)

½ teaspoon Chinese five-spice powder

1 to 2 teaspoons avocado oil or coconut oil

8 green onions, sliced, white/light green and dark green parts separated

1 pound lean ground chicken (or ground turkey; we use 93% lean/7% fat)

2 (12-ounce) bags broccoli slaw (or coleslaw mix)

Optional toppings:

Sesame seeds, Sriracha, sliced avocado, and/or chopped fresh cilantro leaves

Tips from the Dietitians

If prepping this recipe ahead, portion each serving in individual microwave-safe containers.

To reheat in the microwave: Microwave for 60 seconds, then stir. If the food is not hot, microwave for 30 seconds at a time until hot to the touch.

When our brains are craving takeout but our bodies are asking for vegetables, this dish is always the first to come to mind. We transformed our favorite egg rolls by ditching the wrappers and deep fryer, then bumped up the veggies to make them into healthy bowls. Ground chicken or turkey stands in for the usual roast pork and shrimp in egg rolls, and packaged broccoli slaw takes the place of the usual cabbage, carrots, and celery. Not only does it cut down on the prep time, the broccoli slaw is packed with vitamin C and fiber. Anytime we can get the flavor of takeout in a healthy, quick meal we consider that a major win.

In a small bowl, combine the coconut aminos, sesame oil, rice vinegar, garlic, ginger, and five-spice powder. Whisk to combine and then set aside.

Place a large skillet over medium heat. When hot, add the avocado oil and swirl to coat the bottom. Add the white and light green parts of the green onions and cook, stirring occasionally, until the onions start to soften, 2 to 3 minutes.

Add the chicken to the skillet, break it up with a large wooden spoon, and cook, stirring occasionally, until the chicken is cooked through and no longer pink, 5 to 6 minutes. Increase the heat to medium high. Add the broccoli slaw and sauce. Cook, stirring occasionally, until the slaw is crisp-tender, 6 to 7 minutes, or cooked to your liking. Stir in the dark green parts of the green onions, then remove the skillet from the heat.

Serve in bowls, and garnish with sesame seeds, Sriracha, sliced avocado, and/or cilantro leaves, if desired.

Store leftovers in an airtight container in the refrigerator for up to 3 days.

Nutrition Info: (Serving size: 2 cups without the optional toppings) 299 calories, 16g total fat, 3g saturated fat, 665mg sodium, 15g carbs, 9g sugar, 3g fiber, 23g protein

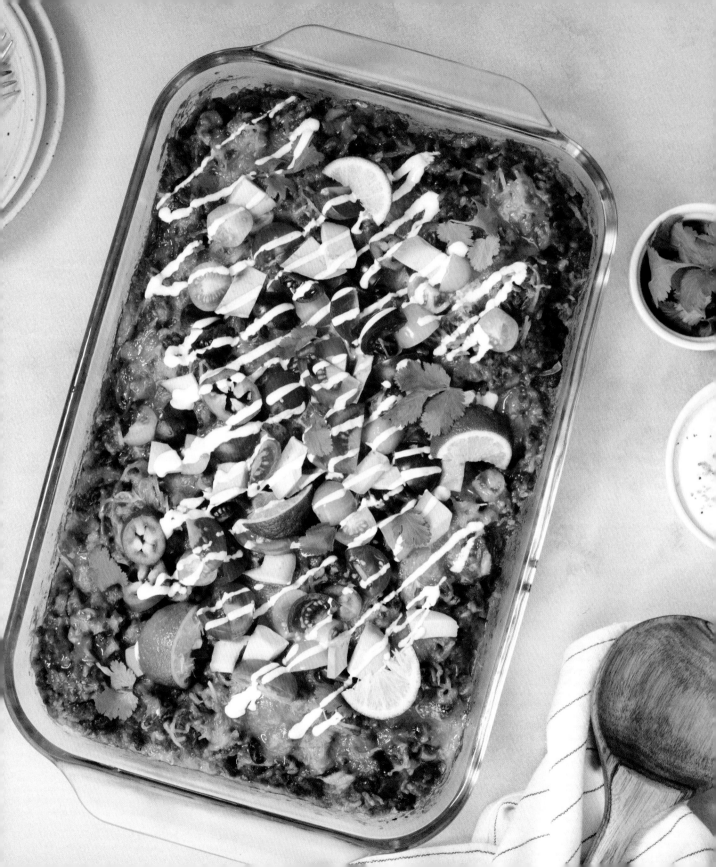

turkey taco casserole

Prep Time: **20 minutes** | Cook Time: **1 hour 15 minutes** | Total Time: **1 hour 35 minutes** | Makes **8 servings**

GF
EF
NF
NAS

FOR THE CASSEROLE

Nonstick cooking spray

2 teaspoons avocado oil or extra-virgin olive oil

2 pounds ground turkey (we use 93% lean/7% fat)

½ medium onion, diced (¾ cup)

1 small bell pepper, diced (any color; ¾ cup)

Fine salt and ground black pepper

1 medium zucchini, diced (1½ cups)

4 garlic cloves, minced

2¾ cups low-sodium chicken broth

1 (14-ounce) can fire-roasted diced tomatoes with their juices

1 (6-ounce) can tomato paste

1½ tablespoons chili powder

1½ teaspoons ground cumin

¾ teaspoon garlic powder

½ teaspoon onion powder

½ teaspoon dried oregano

½ teaspoon paprika

1 (15-ounce) can black beans, drained and rinsed

¾ cup long-grain white rice (or white basmati rice)

2 cups (8 ounces) shredded cheddar or Mexican blend cheese, divided

FOR THE HOMEMADE CREMA

½ cup sour cream

1 to 2 tablespoons fresh lime juice (½ to 1 medium lime), depending on your desired consistency for the crema

Any night of the week can become Taco Tuesday when you serve this delicious casserole. We've taken all of the best flavors of one of our favorite handheld foods and combined them into one cozy, veggie-filled hot dish (that's upper midwestern speak for "casserole," dontcha know?). We love this casserole topped with big dollops of guacamole and pico de gallo or a simple drizzle of homemade crema.

For the casserole: Preheat the oven to 375°F. Spray a 9×13-inch baking dish with cooking spray and set aside.

Place a large skillet over medium-high heat. When hot, add the avocado oil and swirl to coat the bottom. Add the turkey, onion, and bell pepper. Season with salt and pepper. Cook, stirring occasionally, until the turkey is just barely pink and the onion has started to soften, 7 to 8 minutes.

Add the zucchini and garlic to the turkey mixture and stir. Cook, stirring occasionally, until the zucchini is crisp-tender, 3 to 4 minutes.

Remove the skillet from the heat and pour off any excess fat or liquid, then transfer the turkey and vegetables to the prepared baking dish. Add the broth, diced tomatoes with their juices, tomato paste, chili powder, cumin, garlic powder, onion powder, oregano, paprika, and 1½ teaspoons salt and stir well to combine. Add the black beans and rice and stir again to evenly distribute the rice and beans throughout the mixture.

Tightly cover the baking dish with aluminum foil, place it on a rimmed baking sheet, and bake for 55 minutes. Carefully pull back a corner of the foil and test the rice for doneness. If the rice is tender, proceed to the next step. If the rice is not done yet, cover the dish again and bake for 10 more minutes, or until the rice is done.

Remove the foil from the baking dish. Add 1 cup of the cheese and stir into the casserole. Sprinkle the remaining 1 cup cheese evenly over the top and bake, uncovered, 5 to 10 minutes, or until the cheese is bubbly.

Continued on the next page

Optional toppings:
Loaded Guacamole (page 203) or diced avocado, Six-Ingredient Pico de Gallo (page 263) or store-bought pico de gallo, halved cherry tomatoes, chopped fresh cilantro leaves, lime wedges, and/or fresh or pickled jalapeño slices

Remove the casserole from the oven and allow to stand for 5 minutes.

Meanwhile, make the crema: In a small bowl, combine the sour cream with 1 tablespoon of the lime juice. Mix well. If desired, stir in 1 more tablespoon lime juice to achieve a drizzly consistency.

Serve the casserole with the crema and your desired toppings.

Store leftovers in an airtight container in the refrigerator for up to 4 days or in the freezer for up to 3 months.

Nutrition Info: (Serving size: ⅛ of the recipe or 1½ cups with 1 tablespoon crema, without the optional toppings) 436 calories, 23g total fat, 10g saturated fat, 994mg sodium, 22g carbs, 7g sugar, 7g fiber, 38g protein

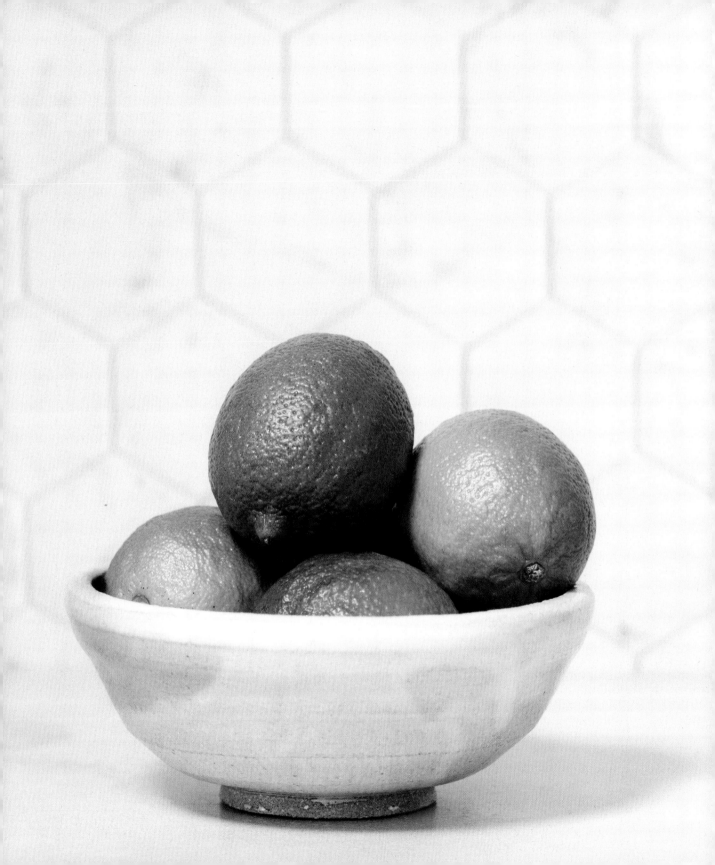

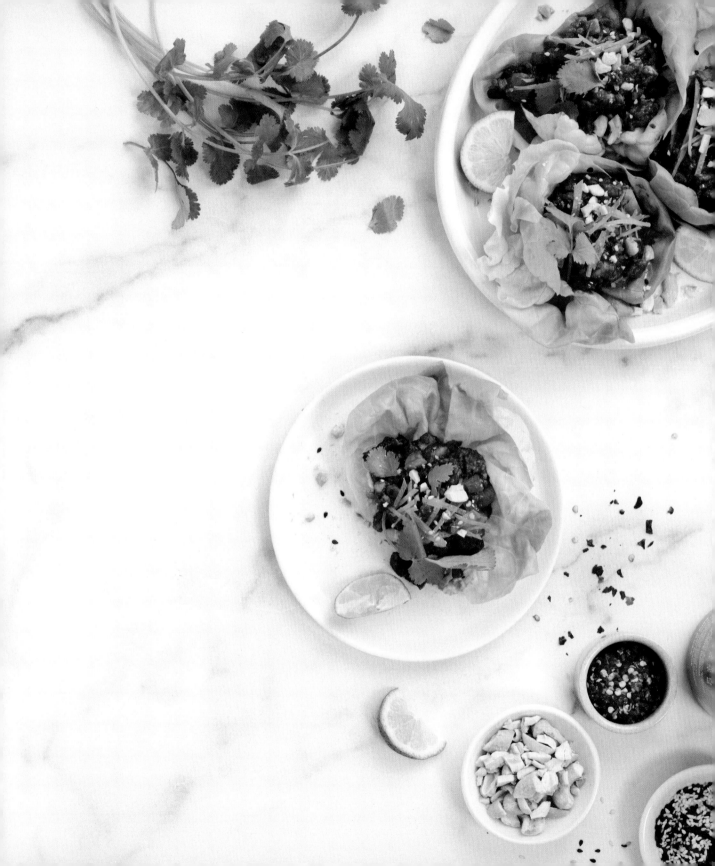

turkey-mushroom lettuce wraps

Prep Time: **20 minutes** | Cook Time: **15 minutes** | Total Time: **35 minutes** | Makes **4 servings**

GF
GrF
DF
EF
NFO
NAS

⅓ cup coconut aminos

3 tablespoons tomato paste

2 tablespoons rice vinegar

1 tablespoon toasted sesame oil

2 garlic cloves, minced

1 teaspoon grated peeled fresh ginger

1 tablespoon avocado or extra-virgin olive oil

1 pound ground turkey (we use 93% lean/7% fat)

8 ounces cremini or button mushrooms, diced (2 cups)

½ medium yellow onion, diced (¾ cup)

Fine salt and ground black pepper

1 (8-ounce) can water chestnuts, drained and diced

1 head butter lettuce or green leaf lettuce, leaves separated

Optional toppings:

Quick-Pickled Carrots or Cucumbers (page 267), shredded cabbage, sliced green onions, chopped fresh cilantro leaves, roughly chopped roasted cashews (omit for nut-free), sesame seeds, crushed red pepper flakes, Sriracha, and/or lime wedges

One thing that we love about this savory turkey and mushroom mixture studded with crunchy water chestnuts is that it can be mounded into cool, crisp lettuce leaves or served over rice for a heartier option. This recipe is a soy-free take on the popular lettuce wraps from P.F. Chang's. Our Coconut-Lime Rice (page 71) makes the perfect base for an epic bowl that you can further top with chopped lettuce, our quick-pickled cucumbers or carrots, sliced avocado, and any of the optional toppings listed for the wraps.

In a small bowl, combine the coconut aminos, tomato paste, vinegar, sesame oil, garlic, and ginger. Whisk well to combine.

Place a large skillet over medium-high heat. When hot, add the avocado oil and swirl to coat the bottom. Add the turkey, mushrooms, and onion. Season with salt and pepper. Break up the turkey with a wooden spoon and cook, stirring occasionally, until the turkey is almost cooked through, 4 to 5 minutes. Add the water chestnuts and continue to cook, stirring occasionally, until the turkey is cooked through, 3 to 4 minutes.

Decrease the heat to medium low. Add the sauce to the skillet and bring to a slow simmer. Continue to cook, stirring occasionally, until the sauce is mostly absorbed, 5 to 7 minutes. Add salt and pepper to taste.

Spoon the turkey-mushroom mixture into the lettuce leaves, layering two leaves if they are small, and serve with your desired toppings.

Store leftover turkey-mushroom filling in an airtight container in the refrigerator for up to 4 days.

Nutrition Info: (Serving size: ¼ of the recipe without the optional toppings) 313 calories, 15g total fat, 3g saturated fat, 475mg sodium, 20g carbs, 10g sugar, 2g fiber, 23g protein

grilled feta-spinach turkey burgers

Prep Time: **15 minutes** | Cook Time: **20 minutes** | Total Time: **35 minutes** | Makes **4 servings**

2 teaspoons avocado oil or
   extra-virgin olive oil, plus more
   for greasing (or use nonstick
   cooking spray)
3 cups loosely packed baby
   spinach, roughly chopped
   (3 ounces)
3 garlic cloves, minced
1 pound ground turkey (we use
   93% lean/7% fat)
⅓ cup crumbled feta cheese
   (omit for dairy-free)
1½ teaspoons dried Italian
   seasoning
½ teaspoon fine salt
¼ teaspoon ground black pepper
¼ teaspoon crushed red pepper
   flakes
Nonstick cooking spray
4 gluten-free hamburger buns,
   butter lettuce or green leaf
   lettuce leaves, or salad greens,
   for serving

Optional toppings:
Quick-Pickled Onions (page 265),
   sliced tomatoes, feta crumbles
   (omit for dairy-free), tzatziki (see
   page 103), and/or your favorite
   burger fixings

Get ready to take a bite out of the most flavorful, juicy grilled burger. There's nothing dry, blah, or bland about these turkey burgers. The Mediterranean seasonings make them especially tasty, while the spinach and feta in the patties keep them from drying out. We like to serve them tucked into lettuce wraps or over a bed of salad greens, topped with fresh tomatoes, pickled onions, and a big dollop of tzatziki sauce.

Preheat the grill to high heat, 425°F to 450°F. If you do not have a grill, use a grill pan on the stovetop over high heat.

Place a small skillet over medium heat. When hot, add the avocado oil and swirl to coat the bottom. Add the spinach and garlic. Cook, stirring occasionally, until the spinach is wilted, 2 to 3 minutes. Remove from the heat and let cool slightly.

In a medium bowl, combine the turkey, spinach, garlic, feta, Italian seasoning, salt, black pepper, and crushed red pepper flakes. Spray your hands with a little cooking spray and form the turkey mixture into four large patties.

Add a small amount of oil or cooking spray to a folded paper towel. Holding the paper towel with tongs, rub it on the hot grill grate or grill pan to grease it. Grill the patties for 10 minutes on one side. Flip and grill until cooked through and an instant-read thermometer inserted into the center of a patty registers 165°F, 6 to 8 minutes.

Serve the patties in the buns or lettuce leaves, or over a bed of salad greens, with your desired toppings.

Store leftover patties in an airtight container in the refrigerator for up to 4 days or in the freezer for up to 2 months.

Nutrition Info: (Serving size: 1 patty without the bun and optional toppings) 223 calories, 13g total fat, 4g saturated fat, 522mg sodium, 2g carbs, 0g sugar, 1g fiber, 23g protein

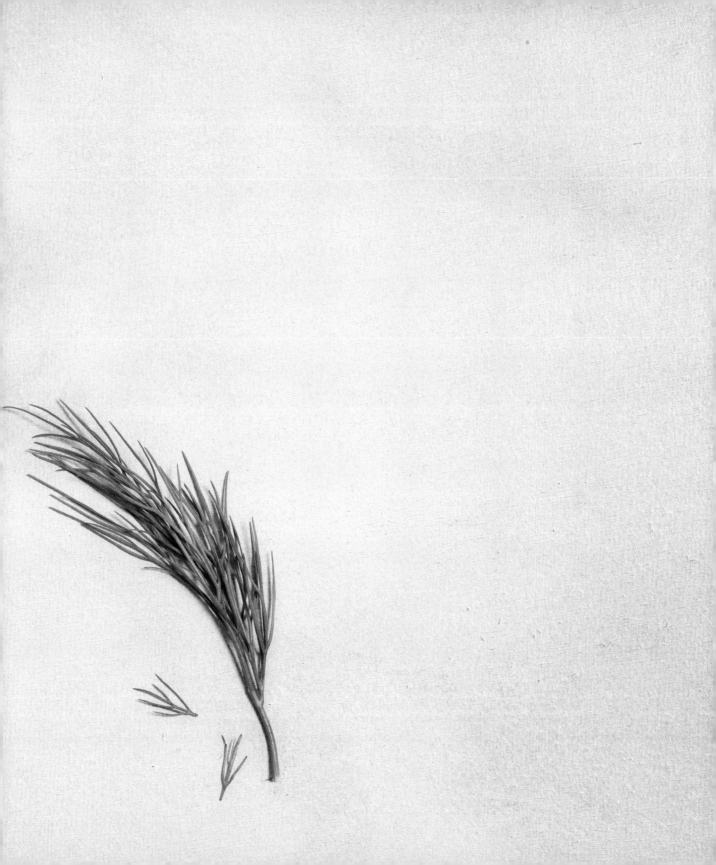

beef & pork entrées

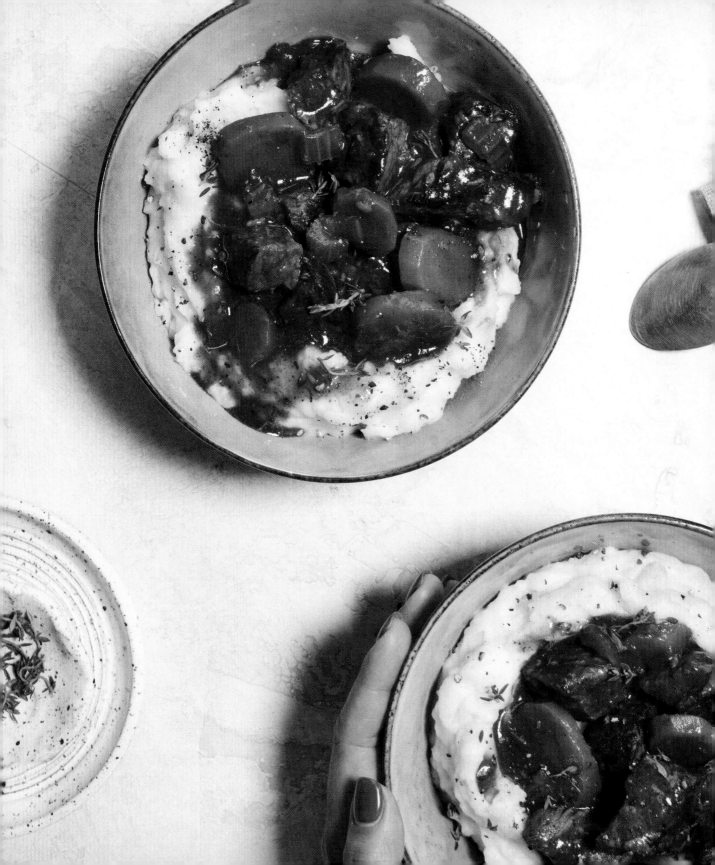

slow cooker irish beef stew

Prep Time: **30 minutes** | Cook Time: **8 hours** | Total Time: **8 hours 30 minutes** | Makes **6 servings**

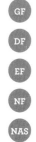

2¼ pounds boneless beef chuck
roast, trimmed of excess fat and
cut into ¾-inch cubes

Fine salt and ground black pepper

6 teaspoons avocado oil or extra-
virgin olive oil, divided

1 large yellow onion, diced
(2½ cups)

1 cup low-sodium beef broth,
divided

4 garlic cloves, minced

4 medium carrots, peeled and
sliced ¼ inch thick (1½ cups)

3 celery stalks, thinly sliced
(¾ cup)

1 (15- to 16-ounce) can gluten-
free stout beer of choice or
2 cups low-sodium beef broth

¼ cup tomato paste

2 bay leaves

1 teaspoon dried thyme

2 tablespoons cornstarch
(optional)

2 tablespoons water, if using
cornstarch

Instant Pot Garlic Mashed
Potatoes (page 62)

Optional garnishes:
Chopped fresh parsley and/or
fresh thyme leaves

Our version of this classic dish is rich and flavorful thanks to gluten-free stout beer, beef broth, and low and slow cooking. The stew is filled with tender hunks of beef and vegetables that just beg to be served over fluffy garlic mashed potatoes for the ultimate soul-warming, budget-friendly comfort food.

Pat the beef dry with paper towels, then season with salt and pepper.

Place a large heavy-bottomed skillet or pot over medium-high heat. When hot, add 2 teaspoons of the avocado oil and swirl to coat the bottom. Add half of the beef in a single layer and cook until well browned, about 2 minutes per side. Transfer to a 6-quart slow cooker. Repeat with 2 more teaspoons of the oil and the remaining beef.

To the same skillet (no need to wipe it out first), add the remaining 2 teaspoons oil and decrease the heat to medium. Add the onion and ½ cup of the beef broth. Cook, scraping up any browned bits from the bottom of the skillet with a wooden spoon, until the onion starts to soften, 8 to 9 minutes. Add the garlic and cook, stirring occasionally, for about 1 minute.

Transfer the onion and garlic to the slow cooker. Add the carrots, celery, beer, tomato paste, bay leaves, thyme, and remaining ½ cup broth and stir to combine. Cover and cook on low for 8 hours.

If desired, thicken the stew with cornstarch: Select the sauté function on the slow cooker, if yours has one, or transfer the stew to a Dutch oven and bring to a simmer over medium-high heat. In a small bowl, whisk the cornstarch with the water to create a thick slurry. Stir into the hot stew and cook, stirring occasionally, for 10 minutes. Add salt and pepper to taste.

Serve over Instant Pot Garlic Mashed Potatoes. Garnish with chopped fresh parsley, if desired. Store any leftovers in separate airtight containers in the refrigerator for up to 4 days or in the freezer for up to 3 months.

Nutrition Info: (Serving size: 1 cup stew plus ¾ cup mashed potatoes, without the optional ingredients) 448 calories, 17g total fat, 7g saturated fat, 225mg sodium, 34g carbs, 6g sugar, 4g fiber, 37g protein

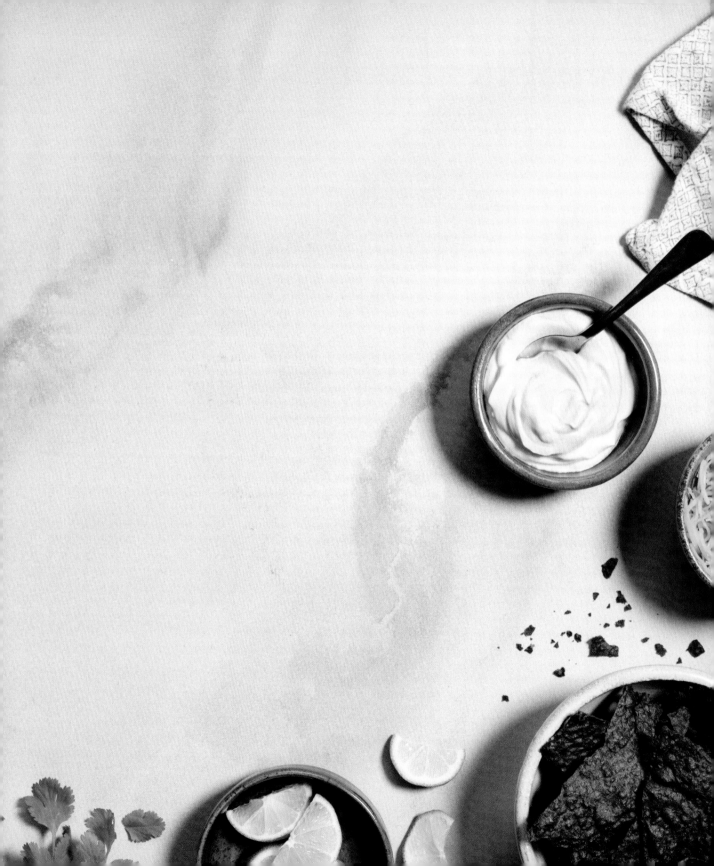

slow cooker game day chili

Prep Time: **20 minutes** | Cook Time: **8 hours** | Total Time: **8 hours 20 minutes** |
Makes **8 servings (about 15 cups)**

GF
GrF
DF
EF
NF
NAS

1 tablespoon avocado oil or extra-virgin olive oil

1 (2-pound) boneless beef chuck roast, trimmed of excess fat and cut into 1-inch cubes (see Tips)

2 (28-ounce) cans fire-roasted diced tomatoes with their juices

2 (15-ounce) cans pinto beans, drained and rinsed

2 (4-ounce) cans diced green chiles with their liquid

1 cup low-sodium beef broth

3 ounces tomato paste

1 medium yellow onion, diced (1½ cups)

1 medium green bell pepper, diced (1 cup)

6 garlic cloves, minced

1 small jalapeño, seeds and membranes removed, finely minced

3 tablespoons chili powder

1 tablespoon ground cumin

1 tablespoon unsweetened cocoa powder

¼ teaspoon chipotle powder

½ teaspoon fine salt, plus more as needed

½ teaspoon ground black pepper, plus more as needed

Optional toppings:
Chopped fresh cilantro leaves, diced avocado, sour cream (omit for dairy-free), shredded cheese (omit for dairy free), crushed tortilla chips (use grain-free version or omit for a grain-free), and/or lime wedges

This recipe is a crowd-pleasing "pull out all the stops" kind of chili. The long, slow-cooking time results in a chili that's thick and concentrated with incredibly rich flavors. We like to set out the chili with a variety of topping options in individual bowls and let family and friends top their bowls however they please.

Place a large skillet or Dutch oven over medium-high heat. When hot, add ½ tablespoon of the avocado oil and swirl to coat the bottom. Add half of the beef in a single layer and cook until well browned, about 2 minutes per side. Transfer to a 6-quart slow cooker. Repeat with the remaining ½ tablespoon oil and beef.

To the slow cooker, add the tomatoes with their juices, beans, green chiles with their liquid, broth, tomato paste, onion, bell pepper, garlic, jalapeño, chili powder, cumin, cocoa powder, chipotle powder, salt, and black pepper and stir well to combine.

Cover the slow cooker and cook on low for 8 to 10 hours. Add more salt and pepper to taste.

Serve the chili with your desired toppings. Store any leftovers in an airtight container in the refrigerator for up to 4 days or in the freezer for up to 3 months.

Tips from the Dietitians
Lean ground beef can be substituted for the beef chuck roast if that's what you have on hand and want to save yourself a trip to the store.

Nutrition Info: (Serving size: 1¾ cups without the optional toppings) 335 calories, 9g total fat, 3g saturated fat, 928mg sodium, 33g carbs, 10g sugar, 11g fiber, 29g protein

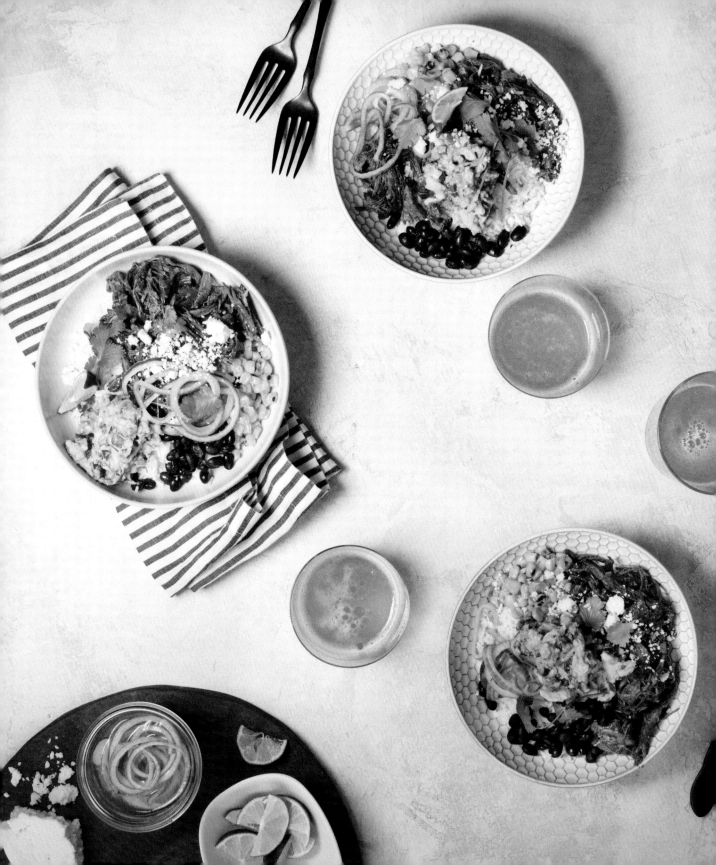

instant pot beef barbacoa burrito bowls

Prep Time: **20 minutes** | Cook Time: **1 hour 15 minutes** | Total Time: **2 hours 5 minutes, includes 30 minutes for pressure buildup and natural release** | Makes **6 servings**

1 (2½-pound) boneless beef chuck roast, trimmed of excess fat and patted dry

1 teaspoon fine salt, plus more as needed

1 tablespoon avocado oil or extra-virgin olive oil

½ medium yellow onion, quartered

6 garlic cloves

¾ cup water

3 tablespoons tomato paste

2 tablespoons fresh lime juice (1 medium lime)

1 tablespoon ground cumin

1 tablespoon dried oregano

Pinch of ground cloves

3 bay leaves

Cooked rice or cauliflower rice, for serving

Optional toppings:

Cooked or canned corn kernels, cooked or canned black beans, shredded lettuce, salsa or Six-Ingredient Pico de Gallo (page 263), Quick-Pickled Onions (page 265), Loaded Guacamole (page 203), chopped fresh cilantro leaves, sour cream (omit for dairy-free), crumbled cotija cheese (omit for dairy-free), and/or lime wedges

When on the road we often stop by a popular fast-casual restaurant for burrito bowls because they're quick, easy, and satisfying. That was the inspiration for these simple, budget-friendly, irresistible bowls that can feed a crowd (or a family for dinner with enough for leftovers). Using the Instant Pot significantly speeds up the cooking time of the barbacoa, which traditionally requires a long cooking process. So now with just twenty minutes of prep time, a little planning, and several options for toppings, restaurant-style burrito bowls can be on the menu any day of the week.

Place the roast on a plate and rub the salt over the surface of the meat.

Select the sauté function on a 6-quart Instant Pot. When the pot is hot, add the avocado oil. Place the roast in the pot and cook until browned, about 2 minutes per side. Press cancel on the Instant Pot.

While the roast is browning, combine the onion, garlic, water, tomato paste, lime juice, cumin, oregano, and cloves in a blender and blend until smooth. Pour over the roast in the Instant Pot, lifting the roast with tongs to allow the sauce to get underneath it.

Top the roast with the bay leaves. Lock the lid in place and switch the valve to the "sealing" position. Set the Instant Pot to cook at high pressure for 75 minutes. (It will take about 10 minutes for the Instant Pot to build up the pressure before the timer starts counting down.)

When the timer goes off, allow the pressure to naturally release for 20 minutes, then switch the vent valve to "venting" to release any residual steam.

Using a slotted spoon, carefully remove the meat and onions to a clean plate. Shred the meat with 2 forks and add 2 to 3 tablespoons of the cooking liquid to taste. Add more salt to taste.

Continued on the next page

Serve the barbacoa in bowls over cooked rice with your desired toppings.

Store leftovers in an airtight container in the refrigerator for up to 4 days or in the freezer for up to 3 months.

> ### Tips from the Dietitians
> No Instant Pot? No problem. Brown the beef in a large skillet or Dutch oven over medium-high heat, then place in a slow cooker along with the sauce. Cook on low for 8 to 10 hours.

Nutrition Info: (Serving size: 4 ounces of the beef barbacoa without rice and the optional toppings) 278 calories, 12g total fat, 5g saturated fat, 442mg sodium, 6g carbs, 3g sugar, 1g fiber, 37g protein

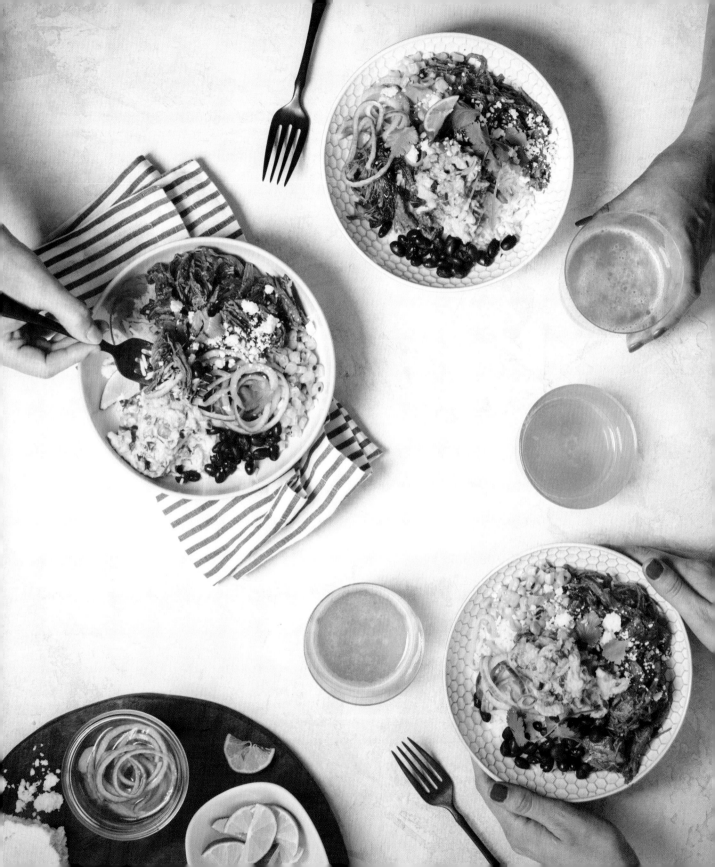

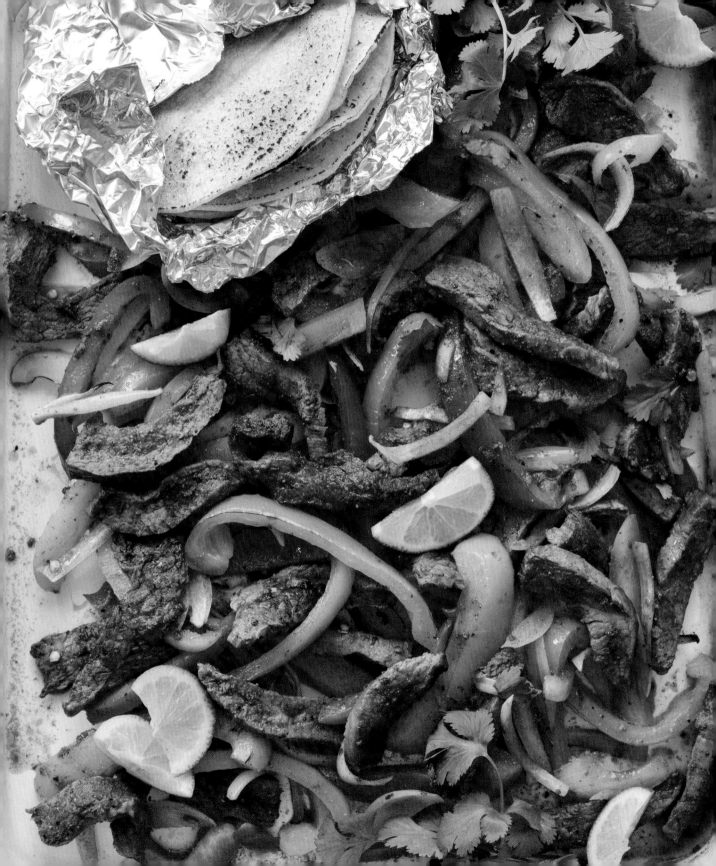

sheet pan steak fajitas

Prep Time: **15 minutes** | Cook Time: **15 minutes** | Total Time: **30 minutes** | Makes **4 servings**

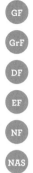

1½ tablespoons avocado oil or extra-virgin olive oil

1 tablespoon fresh lime juice (½ medium lime)

2 teaspoons chili powder

1 teaspoon garlic powder

1 teaspoon ground cumin

½ teaspoon dried oregano

1 teaspoon fine salt

¼ teaspoon ground black pepper

Pinch or two of cayenne pepper (optional)

1 pound flank steak, patted dry, sliced lengthwise, then sliced crosswise into ¼-inch-thick strips (see Tips)

3 medium bell peppers, thinly sliced (any color; 4 cups)

½ medium onion, thinly sliced (1¼ cups)

8 corn tortillas (use grain-free tortillas or cauliflower rice for grain-free)

Optional toppings:

Six-Ingredient Pico de Gallo (page 263), shredded cheese (omit for dairy-free), sour cream (omit for dairy-free), hot sauce of choice, chopped fresh cilantro leaves, and/or lime wedges

This is the perfect busy weeknight meal: It relies on hands-off cooking in the oven, it's on the table in thirty minutes, and has minimal cleanup. It doesn't get any easier than this! We've packed these fajitas with extra bell peppers but kept the spices mild to make it family friendly.

Preheat the oven to 425°F. Line a rimmed baking sheet with parchment paper and set aside.

In a small bowl, combine the avocado oil, lime juice, chili powder, garlic powder, cumin, oregano, salt, and black pepper. Add the cayenne pepper, if desired, for spicier fajitas and stir to combine.

Transfer the steak, bell peppers, and onion to the prepared baking sheet. Drizzle with the oil mixture, and using your hands or tongs, toss to coat. Spread the steak and vegetables in a single layer.

Roast in the oven for 11 to 12 minutes, or until the steak is done to your liking and the vegetables are just tender.

To warm the tortillas, place a large skillet over medium-high heat. When hot, add one to two tortillas and cook 30 seconds per side. Transfer the tortillas to a plate and cover with a clean kitchen towel to keep them warm. Repeat with the remaining tortillas.

Serve the fajitas immediately with the warm tortillas and your desired toppings. Store leftovers in an airtight container in the refrigerator for up to 3 days.

> **Tips from the Dietitians**
> To make the steak easier to slice, wrap it in parchment paper and place it in the freezer for 30 minutes before slicing.

Nutrition Info: (Serving size: ¼ of the recipe without the optional toppings) 404 calories, 16g total fat, 5g saturated fat, 707mg sodium, 35g carbs, 9g sugar, 6g fiber, 30g protein

grilled beef kebabs

Prep Time: **15 minutes** | Cook Time: **10 minutes** | Total Time: **25 minutes, plus 30 minutes for marinating** | Makes **4 servings**

FOR THE KEBABS

1¼ pounds sirloin steak, trimmed and cut into 1-inch cubes

Avocado oil, extra-virgin olive oil, or nonstick cooking spray, for greasing

1 small red onion, cut into 1-inch pieces

2 medium bell peppers, any color, cut into 1-inch pieces

FOR THE MARINADE

2 tablespoons coconut aminos

2 tablespoons red wine vinegar

1 tablespoon Worcestershire sauce

½ teaspoon garlic powder

½ teaspoon dried Italian seasoning

¼ teaspoon fine salt

¼ teaspoon ground black pepper

Tips from the Dietitians

To prep the kebabs ahead, store the marinade, steak, and vegetables in separate airtight containers in the refrigerator for up to 2 days. Marinate the steak for up to 8 hours in the refrigerator.

Sometimes simple is the best way to go. Just steak, onions, peppers, and a pantry-based marinade are all you need to make these tender, juicy kebabs. They can be prepped ahead to grill when you're ready for an easy meal. We love to serve them on a big bed of salad greens with our favorite dressing, like Dairy-Free Ranch Dressing and Dip (page 254) or Honey Mustard Dressing and Dipping Sauce (page 259), but they're also great when served with a side of Baked Sweet Potato Fries with Chipotle-Lime Aioli (page 65).

Place the steak in a shallow bowl and set aside.

Make the marinade: In a small bowl, combine the coconut aminos, vinegar, Worcestershire sauce, garlic powder, Italian seasoning, salt, and pepper and whisk. Pour over the steak and allow to marinate for at least 30 minutes (and up to 8 hours) in the refrigerator.

Grill the kebabs: Add a small amount of avocado oil or cooking spray to a folded paper towel. Holding the paper towel with tongs, rub it on the grill grate to grease it. Preheat the grill to medium-high heat (375°F to 400°F).

Thread the steak, onion, and bell pepper pieces onto four metal skewers, alternating the ingredients as you go. Discard the marinade.

Place the kebabs directly on the grill grate and cook 4 to 5 minutes per side or until done to your liking.

Store leftovers, removed from the skewers, in an airtight container in the refrigerator for up to 3 days.

Nutrition Info: (Serving size: ¼ of the recipe) 179 calories, 5g total fat, 2g saturated fat, 244mg sodium, 9g carbs, 6g sugar, 2g fiber, 26g protein

slow cooker tacos al pastor

Prep Time: **20 minutes** | Cook Time: **8 hours** | Total Time: **8 hours 20 minutes** | Makes **8 servings**

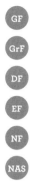

1 (3- to 3½-pound) boneless pork shoulder roast, trimmed of excess fat and cut into 2-inch pieces

4 cups finely diced fresh pineapple (about 1 medium pineapple), divided

½ medium white onion, quartered

6 garlic cloves

5 tablespoons tomato paste

¼ cup fresh lime juice (2 small limes)

2 tablespoons apple cider vinegar

2 tablespoons chili powder

1 teaspoon ground cumin

¾ teaspoon chipotle powder (see Tips)

½ teaspoon fine salt, plus more as needed

16 corn tortillas (use grain-free tortillas or cauliflower rice for grain-free)

1 cup loosely packed fresh cilantro leaves, roughly chopped

Optional for serving:

Finely diced white onion or Quick-Pickled Onions (page 265), Loaded Guacamole, and/or Cilantro-Lime Slaw

Tips from the Dietitians

If you like your tacos with a little more spice, increase the chipotle powder.

If you asked Jessica to name her favorite food, she'd tell you, "Tacos. Without a doubt, tacos." She'd rather track down a roadside taco stand or truck than dine in the fanciest of restaurants. Wherever she travels in the Southwest or Mexico, tacos al pastor with their sweet and spicy pork, juicy pineapple, crunchy raw onions, and bright, fresh cilantro are a must. This recipe is her homemade fix for those times between travels when the siren call for tacos is too hard to resist. These tacos are delicious served with a side of our Cilantro-Lime Slaw (page 58) and Loaded Guacamole (page 203).

Add the pork to a 6-quart slow cooker.

In a blender, combine 2 cups of the pineapple with the onion, garlic, tomato paste, lime juice, vinegar, chili powder, cumin, chipotle powder, and salt and blend until smooth. Pour over the pork and stir. Cover the slow cooker and cook on low for 8 hours (or high for 4 hours).

Using a slotted spoon, transfer the pork to a medium bowl or shallow dish, and reserve the cooking liquid. Using two forks, shred the pork into bite-size pieces, then add some of the reserved cooking liquid to the pork, to taste. Add more salt to taste.

To warm the tortillas, place a large skillet over medium-high heat. When hot, add 1 to 2 tortillas and cook 30 seconds per side. Transfer the tortillas to a plate and cover with a clean kitchen towel to keep them warm. Repeat with the remaining tortillas.

To serve, top the warm tortillas with the pork, remaining pineapple, the chopped cilantro, diced white onion, and Loaded Guacamole, if using. Serve with Cilantro-Lime Slaw, if desired.

Store leftovers in an airtight container in the refrigerator for up to 4 days or in the freezer for up to 3 months.

Nutrition Info: (Serving size: two tacos with ¼ cup pineapple, without the optional accompaniments) 364 calories, 11g total fat, 3g saturated fat, 468mg sodium, 31g carbs, 12g sugar, 4g fiber, 36g protein

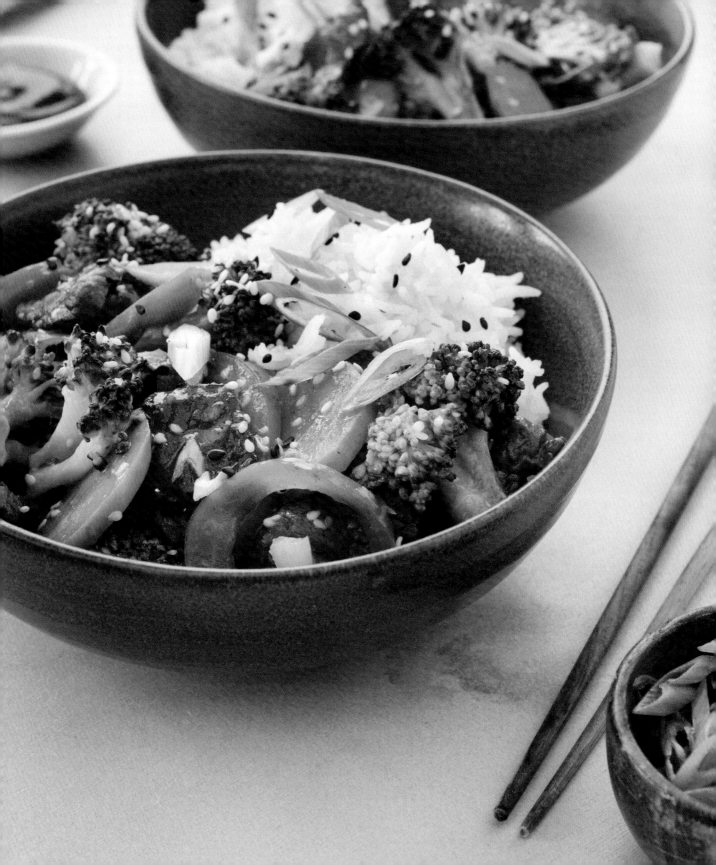

beef & broccoli (& then some!)

Prep Time: **20 minutes** | Cook Time: **15 minutes** | Total Time: **35 minutes** | Makes **4 servings**

GF
GrF
DF
EF
NF

FOR THE SAUCE

⅔ cup coconut aminos

⅓ cup water

2 tablespoons cornstarch (or 3 tablespoons arrowroot starch, for grain-free)

1 tablespoon toasted sesame oil

1 tablespoon honey

3 garlic cloves, minced or grated

1¼ teaspoons grated peeled fresh ginger

FOR THE BEEF AND VEGETABLES

1 tablespoon plus 2 teaspoons avocado oil or extra-virgin olive oil, divided, plus more as needed

2 medium carrots, peeled and thinly sliced on the diagonal (1 cup)

1 medium red bell pepper, thinly sliced (1 cup)

1 pound broccoli, trimmed and cut into bite-size florets (5 to 6 cups)

1 tablespoon water

1 pound flank steak, trimmed, very thinly sliced into bite-size pieces, and patted dry (see Tips)

Optional for serving:

Cooked rice (use cauliflower rice for grain-free), thinly sliced green onions, and/or sesame seeds

This easy-to-make entrée inspired by the Chinese take-out dish is easy on your budget as well. We put our own healthy twist on it by adding carrots and bell peppers to the broccoli for an extra dose of vitamins, fiber, and eye-catching color. We use flank steak, but other cuts such as sirloin, tri-tip, or skirt steak also work well.

Make the sauce: In a small bowl, combine the coconut aminos, water, cornstarch, sesame oil, honey, garlic, and ginger. Whisk well to combine and set aside.

Prepare the beef and vegetables: Place a large skillet over medium-high heat. When hot, add the 2 teaspoons avocado oil and swirl to coat the bottom. Add the carrots and bell pepper and cook, stirring occasionally, for 3 minutes.

Add the broccoli and water to the skillet, cover, and cook until the broccoli is bright green and crisp-tender, about 3 minutes. Uncover and continue to cook 1 minute, stirring constantly. Transfer the vegetables to a plate and return the skillet to medium-high heat (no need to wipe it out).

When hot, add the 1 tablespoon avocado oil to the same skillet and swirl to coat the bottom. When the oil just starts to shimmer, add the beef in a single layer, working in two batches and adding more oil to coat the skillet if necessary. Cook until browned and almost cooked through, 60 to 90 seconds per side. Drain off some of the liquid if there is a lot of it left in the skillet between batches.

Stir the sauce well, then add it to the skillet with all of the beef. Decrease the heat to medium and allow the sauce to simmer until it starts to thicken, about 4 minutes. Return the vegetables to the skillet and toss to combine them with the beef and sauce.

Continued on the next page

Serve over cooked rice and sprinkle with green onions and/or sesame seeds, if desired. Store leftovers in an airtight container in the refrigerator for up to 3 days.

Tips from the Dietitians
To make the steak easier to slice, wrap it in parchment paper and place it in the freezer for 30 minutes before slicing.

Nutrition Info: (Serving size: 1¼ cups without the optional accompaniments) 359 calories, 17g total fat, 5g saturated fat, 796mg sodium, 24g carbs, 15g sugar, 4g fiber, 26g protein

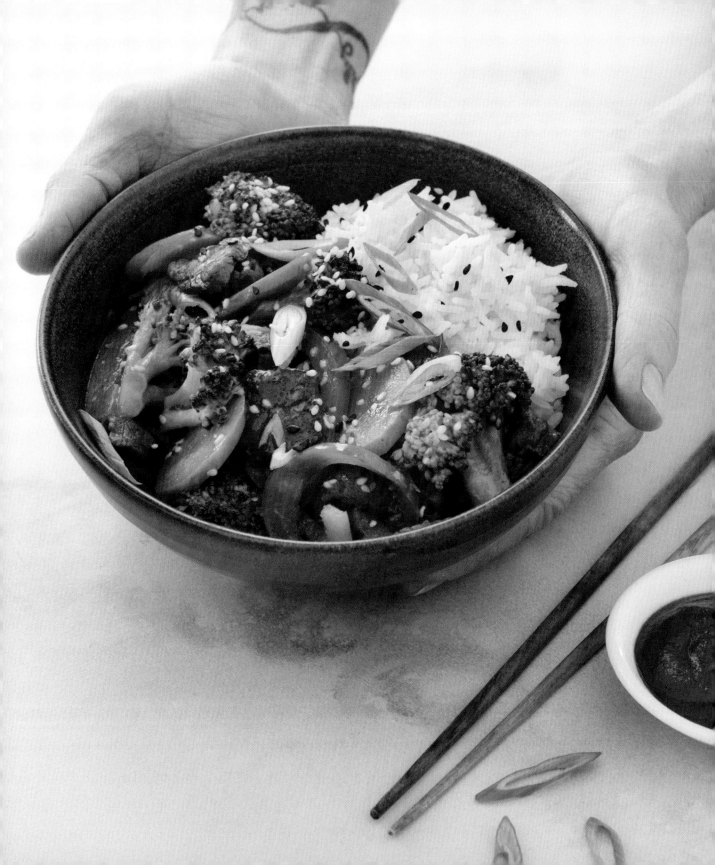

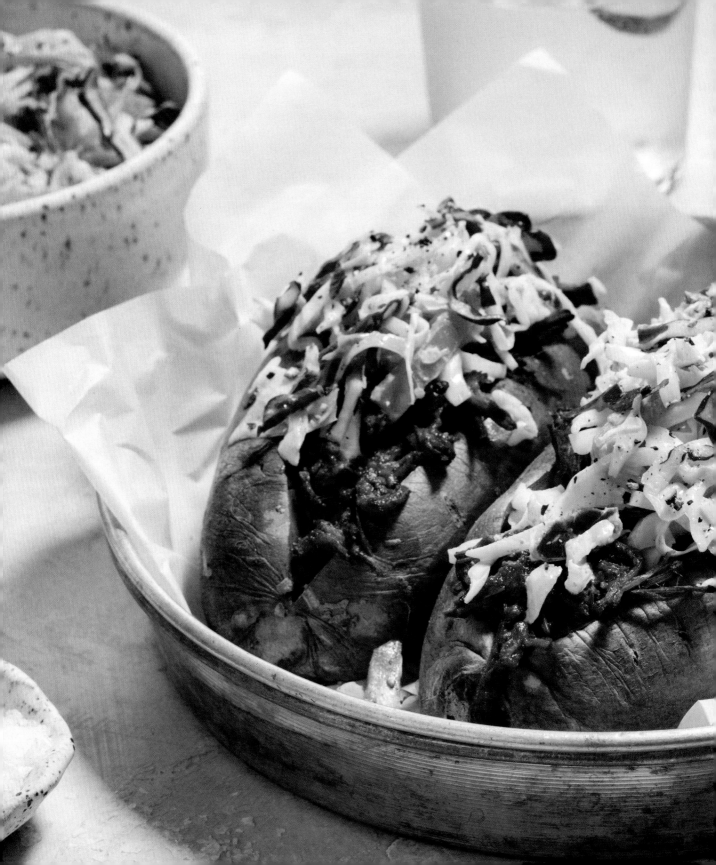

shredded barbecue beef–stuffed sweet potatoes

Prep Time: **20 minutes** | Cook Time: **4 hours 15 minutes** | Total Time: **4 hours 35 minutes** | Makes **8 servings**

GF
GrF
DF
EF
NF
NAS

FOR THE SAUCE
1 (6-ounce) can tomato paste
¼ cup water
2 tablespoons Dijon mustard
2 tablespoons apple cider vinegar
2 teaspoons chili powder
2 teaspoons smoked paprika
¾ teaspoon fine salt
½ teaspoon ground black pepper

FOR THE BEEF
1 (2¾- to 3-pound) boneless beef
   chuck roast, trimmed of excess
   fat and patted dry
Fine salt and ground black pepper
2 tablespoons avocado oil or
   extra-virgin olive oil, divided
1 medium yellow onion, thinly
   sliced
4 garlic cloves, minced
¼ cup water

FOR THE SWEET POTATOES (SEE TIPS)
8 medium sweet potatoes,
   scrubbed clean (5 to 6 pounds)
Avocado oil or extra-virgin olive
   oil, for rubbing
Fine salt

Optional for serving:
Every Occasion Coleslaw
   (page 59)

You can always count on us for healthy comfort food. After all, it is what our blog is known for! This recipe calls for a longer cooking time, but most of that time is hands-off. We also give directions for using the slow cooker so you don't have to leave the oven on if you plan to be out of the house all day. The saucy, tender beef is delicious when stuffed into baked sweet potatoes—especially when topped with creamy, vinegary coleslaw. But it can also be served as a sandwich for a more traditional approach to this American favorite.

Position racks in the center and lower third of the oven and preheat it to 250°F.

Prepare the sauce: In a medium bowl, combine the tomato paste, water, mustard, vinegar, chili powder, paprika, salt, and pepper. Stir to combine and then set aside.

Prepare the beef: Cut the roast crosswise into three equal pieces. Season with salt and pepper.

Place a Dutch oven over medium-high heat. When hot, add 1 tablespoon of the avocado oil and swirl to coat the bottom. Add the beef and cook, flipping once, until browned, 4 to 5 minutes per side. Transfer to a plate.

Keep the Dutch oven over medium-high heat, add the remaining 1 tablespoon oil, and swirl to coat the bottom. Add the onion and garlic and cook, stirring frequently, until the onion starts to soften, about 5 minutes. Add the water to the Dutch oven and use a wooden spoon to scrape up any browned bits. Remove from the heat and stir in the sauce.

Place the beef in the Dutch oven in a single layer. Cover and bake on the center rack for about 4 hours, or until the beef easily shreds with a fork.

After the beef has been in the oven for 2 hours, bake the sweet potatoes: Line a baking sheet with parchment paper. Rub the sweet potatoes with

Continued on the next page

avocado oil and season with salt. While the beef is in the oven, bake the potatoes on the prepared baking sheet on the lower rack for 2 to 2½ hours, or until the potatoes are easily pierced with a fork.

When the beef is done, remove from the oven, shred it with two forks right in the Dutch oven, then stir the shredded meat into the sauce and onions. Add more salt and pepper to taste. Cover and place the Dutch oven over low heat on the stove to keep warm, if the sweet potatoes are not ready yet.

Make a slit lengthwise down the middle of each sweet potato. Using your hands, push the ends of each potato together to create an opening. If the potatoes are too hot to handle, protect your hands with a kitchen towel. Spoon the shredded beef into the opening. Top the beef with Every Occasion Coleslaw, if desired, and serve.

Store leftovers in an airtight container in the refrigerator for up to 4 days. The beef can be stored in the freezer for up to 3 months.

Tips from the Dietitians

Want to make this a set-it-and-forget-it meal? After searing the beef, transfer it to the slow cooker with the sauce, raw onions, and garlic, and cook on low for 8 to 10 hours. Then bake the sweet potatoes according to the directions in the following Tip.

If you are not baking the sweet potatoes at the same time as the beef: Preheat the oven to 375°F and line a baking sheet with parchment paper. Rub the sweet potatoes with oil and season with salt. Bake on the prepared baking sheet for 45 to 60 minutes, or until fork tender.

If baking the sweet potatoes in advance, let them cool, then store them in an airtight container in the refrigerator for up to 3 days. To reheat, place the sweet potatoes on a microwave-safe plate. Make a slit lengthwise down the middle of each potato and microwave for 60 seconds or until hot.

Nutrition Info: (Serving size: 4 ounces of the shredded barbecue beef plus 1 sweet potato, without the coleslaw) 414 calories, 11g total fat, 4g saturated fat, 438mg sodium, 42g carbs, 17g sugar, 8g fiber, 34g protein

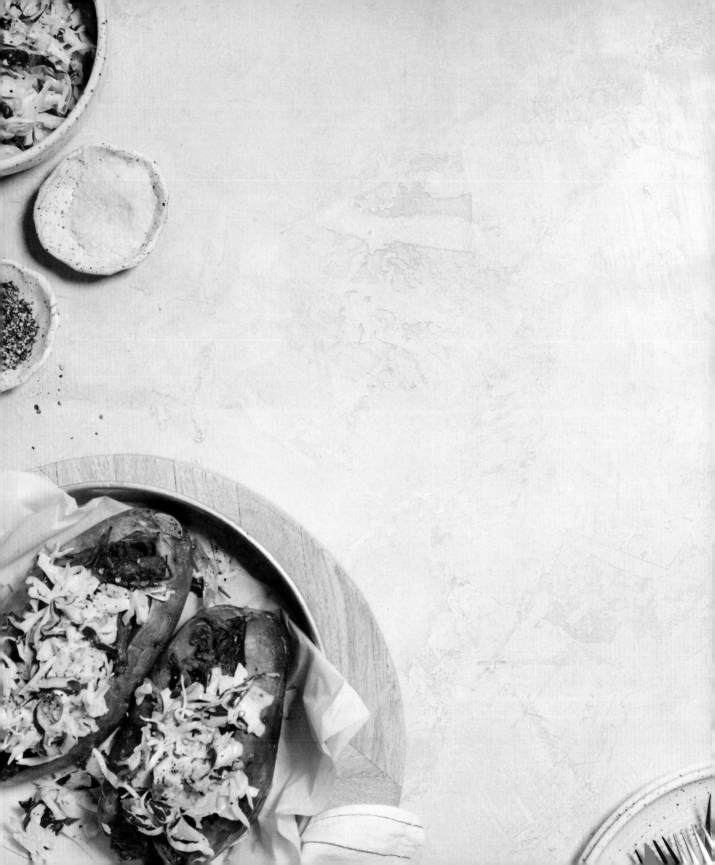

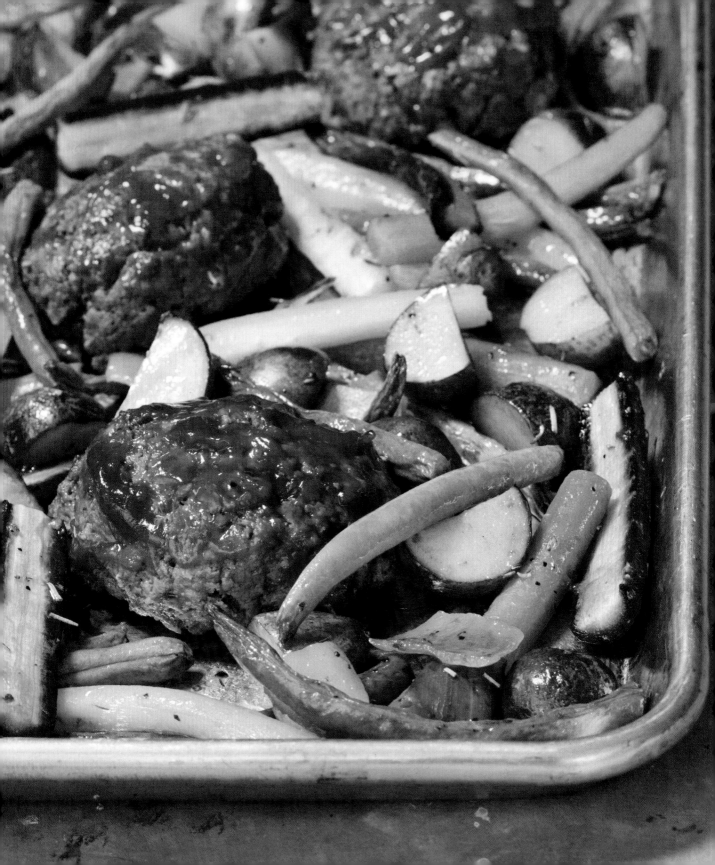

sheet pan mini meat loaf dinner

Prep Time: **25 minutes** | Cook Time: **30 minutes** | Total Time: **55 minutes** | Makes **4 servings**

GF
GrF
DF
EF
NFO
NAS

FOR THE VEGETABLES

12 ounces baby red potatoes, scrubbed clean and halved, or quartered if large (2 to 2½ cups)

12 ounces green beans, trimmed and cut into 2- to 3-inch pieces (3 to 3½ cups)

10 ounces carrots, peeled and cut into ½×2½-inch sticks (1½ to 2 cups)

½ medium red onion, cut into ½- to 1-inch chunks (1 cup)

3 garlic cloves, minced

1 tablespoon avocado oil or extra-virgin olive oil

½ teaspoon dried rosemary

¼ teaspoon dried thyme

¼ teaspoon fine salt

⅛ teaspoon ground black pepper

FOR THE MEAT LOAVES

½ cup ketchup, divided, plus more for serving (optional; see Tips)

1 pound lean ground beef (we use 93% lean/7% fat)

3 tablespoons almond flour (or gluten-free bread crumbs, for nut-free)

2 garlic cloves, minced

½ teaspoon onion powder

¼ teaspoon dried rosemary

¼ teaspoon dried thyme

¼ teaspoon fine salt

Pinch of ground black pepper

Need something hearty and filling for dinner tonight? Try this meat loaf with roasted potatoes and vegetables that cook entirely on a single sheet pan! It's like a Sunday dinner, only much simpler and with far fewer dishes to wash, so it's perfect for any night of the week. Shaping the herbed ground beef into mini loaves significantly shortens the cooking time, enabling you to get dinner on the table faster. Stacie was not always a fan of meat loaf growing up, but this version she created for her family made her a convert. The combination of herbs and garlic along with the perfectly roasted vegetables has made this a regular dish on the menu at her dinner table.

Preheat the oven to 400°F. Line a rimmed baking sheet with parchment paper and set aside.

Roast the vegetables: Place the potatoes, green beans, carrots, onion, and garlic on the prepared baking sheet. Drizzle with the avocado oil and sprinkle with the rosemary, thyme, salt, and pepper. Toss the vegetables to coat evenly with the oil and seasoning. Roast in the oven for 20 minutes.

Meanwhile, make the meat loaves: Reserve ¼ cup of the ketchup for glazing, then place the remaining ¼ cup in a medium bowl. Add the remaining ingredients and mix with clean hands until well combined. Form the mixture into four oblong mini loaves, each ¾ inch thick.

When the 20 minutes are up for the vegetables, remove the baking sheet from the oven, toss the vegetables, and spread them out to clear four spaces for the meat loaves. Place the meat loaves on the baking sheet and brush each with the reserved ketchup.

Bake for 12 to 15 minutes, or until an instant-read thermometer inserted into the center of a loaf reads 165°F.

Continued on the next page

Remove from the oven and serve with ketchup for dipping, if desired.

Store leftovers in an airtight container in the refrigerator for up to 3 days.

Tips from the Dietitians

If you're looking to avoid added sugars, use ketchup that is made without sugar.

Change things up by simply swapping out the ketchup for your favorite barbecue sauce or our Homemade Barbecue Sauce (page 260).

Nutrition Info: (Serving size: ¼ of the recipe or 1 meat loaf plus 1⅓ cups vegetables, without the optional ketchup) 369 calories, 11g total fat, 3g saturated fat, 726mg sodium, 40g carbs, 15g sugar, 8g fiber, 29g protein

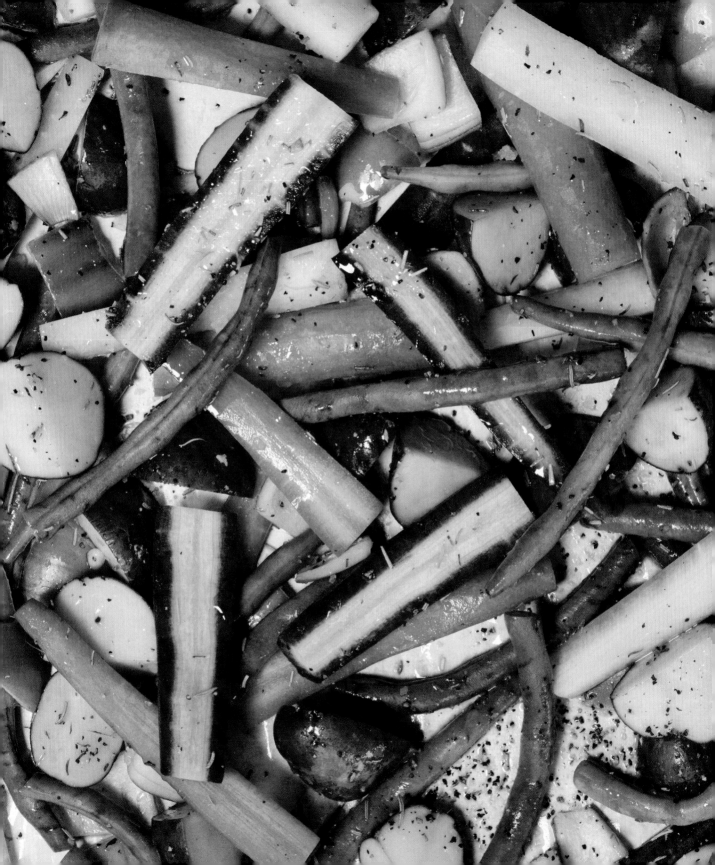

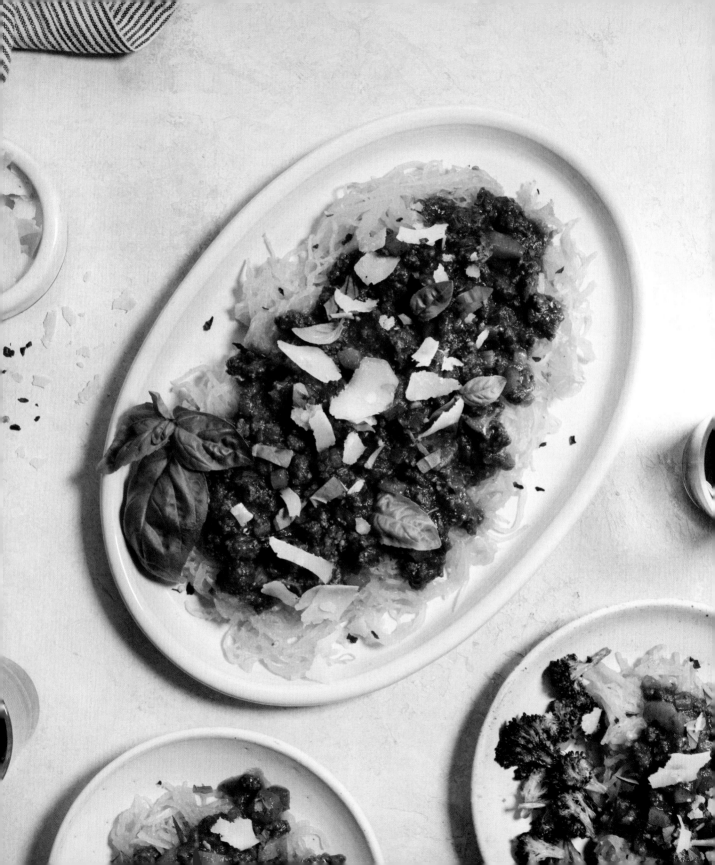

sunday supper beef bolognese sauce

Prep Time: **25 minutes** | Cook Time: **1 hour 5 minutes** | Total Time: **1 hour 30 minutes** | Makes **6 servings**

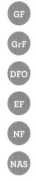

4 bacon slices (4 ounces; see Tips), chopped

1 medium yellow onion, diced (1½ cups)

3 medium carrots, peeled and diced (1½ cups)

3 medium celery stalks, diced (1 cup)

4 garlic cloves, minced

1 pound lean ground beef (we use 93% lean/7% fat)

1 (28-ounce) can tomato sauce

¼ cup water

2 teaspoons dried Italian seasoning

2 teaspoons balsamic vinegar

½ teaspoon fine salt, plus more as needed

¼ teaspoon ground black pepper, plus more as needed

¼ teaspoon crushed red pepper flakes (optional)

FOR SERVING

Cooked gluten-free pasta of choice or Oven-Roasted Spaghetti Squash (page 63)

Freshly grated or shaved Parmesan cheese (omit for dairy-free)

Chopped fresh basil leaves (optional)

Don't let the long cooking time steer you away from this recipe. Most of that time is hands-off for simmering to create a thick, hearty sauce while filling your kitchen with the most inviting, appetite-stimulating aromas. Serve the Bolognese over pasta or strands of roasted spaghetti squash, with a side of Crispy Broccoli (page 70) for the ultimate Sunday supper.

Place a large pot or Dutch oven over medium-high heat. When hot, add the bacon and cook, stirring occasionally, until crispy, 6 to 8 minutes. Pour off all but 1 to 1½ tablespoons of the bacon grease from the pot. Wipe the bacon grease from the side of the pot with a paper towel and return the pot to the stove over medium-high heat.

Add the onion, carrots, and celery to the pot and stir. Cook, stirring occasionally, until the onion starts to soften, 5 to 6 minutes. Add the garlic and beef and break up the meat with a wooden spoon. Cook, stirring occasionally, until the beef is no longer pink, 7 to 8 minutes.

Add the tomato sauce, water, Italian seasoning, vinegar, salt, black pepper, and red pepper flakes, if using, and stir to combine. Bring the sauce to a simmer and cover. Adjust the heat as needed to maintain a gentle simmer, and cook, stirring occasionally, until the sauce is thick and the carrots are tender, about 45 minutes.

Remove the pot from the heat. Add more salt and pepper to taste.

Serve the Bolognese over pasta or Oven-Roasted Spaghetti Squash. Top with Parmesan cheese and/or chopped basil leaves, if desired.

Store leftovers in an airtight container in the refrigerator for up to 4 days or in the freezer for up to 3 months.

Tips from the Dietitians
If you're looking to avoid added sugars, use bacon that is made without sugar.

Nutrition Info: (Serving size: 1 cup sauce without the pasta, squash, and optional accompaniments) 198 calories, 7g total fat, 3g saturated fat, 618mg sodium, 12g carbs, 7g sugar, 3g fiber, 22g protein

easy skillet meatballs & marinara sauce

Prep Time: **10 minutes** | Cook Time: **40 minutes** | Total Time: **50 minutes** | Makes **6 servings**

FOR THE MEATBALLS

2 teaspoons avocado oil or extra-virgin olive oil, divided

3 garlic cloves, minced

4 cups loosely packed spinach, chopped (4 ounces)

1½ pounds lean ground beef (we use 93% lean/7% fat)

1 teaspoon dried Italian seasoning

¾ teaspoon fine salt

¼ teaspoon ground black pepper

FOR THE MARINARA SAUCE

1 teaspoon avocado oil or extra-virgin olive oil

3 garlic cloves, minced

1 (28-ounce) can crushed tomatoes

1 (14-ounce) can tomato sauce

2 tablespoons tomato paste

1½ teaspoons dried Italian seasoning

½ teaspoon fine salt, plus more as needed

¼ teaspoon ground black pepper, plus more as needed

1 teaspoon balsamic vinegar

Pinch of crushed red pepper flakes (optional)

We've never met a kid (or adult, for that matter) who doesn't love a big plate of spaghetti and meatballs. Maybe it's the meatballs, maybe it's the rich, flavorful sauce, or maybe it's all the twirling and slurping of the noodles. We have no idea, we just know that plates are clean when we serve this meal to our own families. While we love noodles, swapping them out for spaghetti squash is an easy way to get more veggies on your plate.

Make the meatballs: Place a large skillet over medium heat. When hot, add 1 teaspoon of the avocado oil and all of the garlic and cook, stirring constantly to avoid burning the garlic, until fragrant, about 30 seconds. Add the spinach and cook, stirring often, until wilted, about 2 minutes. Transfer to a medium bowl and allow the spinach to cool slightly.

To the bowl with the spinach, add the beef, Italian seasoning, salt, and black pepper. Stir to combine, then shape the mixture into 24 balls (about 1 ounce each).

Return the skillet to medium-high heat (no need to wipe it out first). When hot, add the remaining 1 teaspoon avocado oil and the meatballs. Cook until browned and almost cooked through, about 2 minutes per side (or about 12 minutes total). Transfer the meatballs to a plate and set aside.

Make the marinara sauce: Wipe the skillet clean with a paper towel, then place it over medium-low heat. Add the oil and garlic and cook, stirring constantly, until fragrant, about 30 seconds.

To the skillet, add the crushed tomatoes, tomato sauce, tomato paste, Italian seasoning, salt, and black pepper to the skillet and stir well. Increase the heat to medium-high to bring the sauce to a simmer. Stir, then decrease the heat slightly to maintain a gentle simmer. Simmer, uncovered, stirring occasionally, for 15 minutes.

Stir in the balsamic vinegar and red pepper flakes, if using, then return the meatballs to the skillet. Cover and simmer until the meatballs are

Cooked gluten-free pasta of
  choice (use Oven-Roasted
  Spaghetti Squash, page 63, for
  grain-free)
Freshly grated or shaved
  Parmesan cheese (optional;
  omit for dairy-free)
Chopped fresh basil leaves
  (optional)

cooked through and the sauce has thickened, about 15 minutes. Add more salt and pepper to taste.

Serve the meatballs and marinara over pasta or Oven-Baked Spaghetti Squash. Top with Parmesan cheese and/or basil, if desired.

Store leftovers in an airtight container in the refrigerator for up to 4 days.

Nutrition Info: (Serving size: 4 meatballs plus ⅔ cup sauce, without the pasta, squash, and/or optional accompaniments) 237 calories, 6g total fat, 2g saturated fat, 774mg sodium, 16g carbs, 7g sugar, 5g fiber, 29g protein

sloppy joe casserole

Prep Time: **25 minutes** | Cook Time: **35 minutes** | Total Time: **1 hour** | Makes **8 servings**

2 teaspoons avocado oil or extra-virgin olive oil

½ medium yellow onion, diced (1 cup)

½ medium bell pepper, any color, diced (1 cup)

2 pounds lean ground beef (we use 93% lean/7% fat)

3 garlic cloves, minced

1 (6-ounce) can tomato paste

1 cup water

2 tablespoons yellow or Dijon mustard

2 tablespoons coconut aminos

1 tablespoon apple cider vinegar

½ teaspoon smoked paprika

1 teaspoon fine salt, plus more as needed

¼ teaspoon ground black pepper, plus more as needed

Instant Pot Garlic Mashed Potatoes (page 62)

1 cup shredded cheddar cheese (omit for dairy-free)

Classic midwestern comfort foods combine to make this hearty, crave-worthy casserole. When Stacie was growing up, casseroles made a regular appearance on the menu at her home: tater tot, tuna noodle, and chicken and biscuit, to name a few. Her Grandma Verna was known for her sloppy joe recipe, so Stacie decided to turn it into a casserole topped with fluffy mashed potatoes and melted shredded cheddar cheese (per her husband's request). It's a recipe you'll be sure to come back to again and again, midwestern or not! We like it served with a side of Crispy Broccoli (page 70) or steamed green beans.

Preheat the oven to 375°F.

Place a large oven-safe skillet over medium-high heat. (If you don't have a large oven-safe skillet, see Tips.) When hot, add the avocado oil, onion, and bell pepper and cook, stirring occasionally, until the onion starts to soften, 5 to 8 minutes. Add the beef and garlic and break up the meat with a wooden spoon. Cook, stirring occasionally, until the beef is browned and almost cooked through, 10 to 12 minutes.

To the skillet, add the tomato paste, water, mustard, coconut aminos, vinegar, paprika, salt, and black pepper and stir well to combine. Bring to a simmer and cook until the beef is cooked through and the vegetables are tender, 5 to 7 minutes. Add more salt and pepper to taste.

Spoon the mashed potatoes over the meat mixture in six evenly spaced mounds. Spread the potatoes out to cover all but the very edges of the surface. Sprinkle the cheese over the top, if using. Bake for about 10 minutes, or until hot and the edges of the casserole are bubbling.

Remove the casserole from the oven and serve.

Store leftovers in an airtight container in the refrigerator for up to 4 days or in the freezer for up to 3 months.

Tips from the Dietitians

If you don't have a large oven-safe skillet, you can make the sloppy joe filling in a large skillet of any kind. Transfer the filling to a 9×13-inch baking dish coated with cooking spray, then proceed with the recipe as written.

Nutrition Info: (Serving size: about 1¼ cups) 300 calories, 10g total fat, 5g saturated fat, 956mg sodium, 24g carbs, 6g sugar, 4g fiber, 29g protein

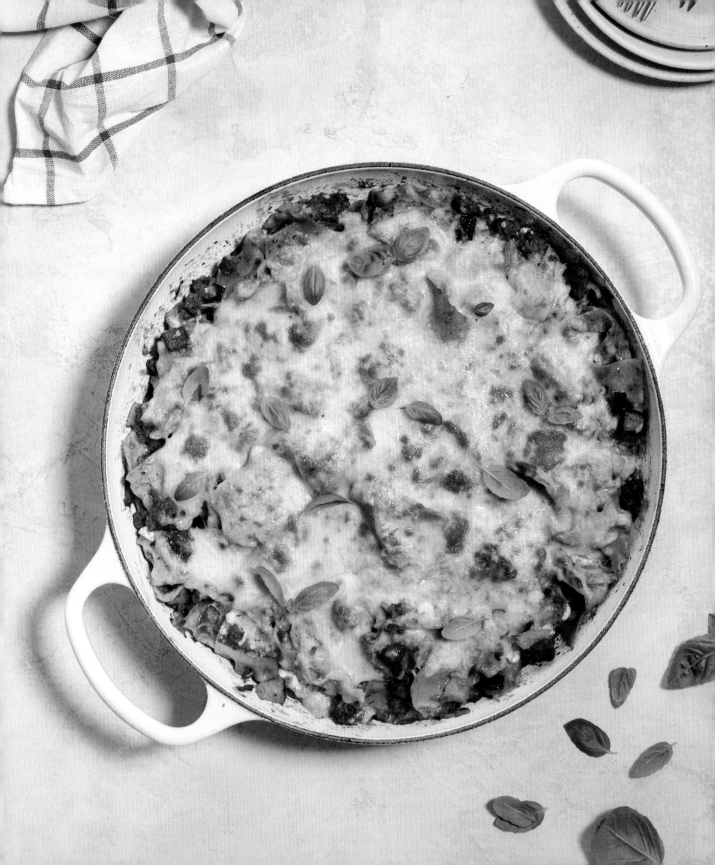

easy skillet lasagna

Prep Time: **15 minutes** | Cook Time: **50 minutes** | Total Time: **1 hour 5 minutes, plus 5 minutes standing time** | Makes **8 servings**

1 teaspoon avocado oil or extra-virgin olive oil

1 pound lean ground beef (we use 93% lean/7% fat)

1 medium zucchini, cut into ¼-inch dice (1½ cups)

1 medium yellow bell pepper, cut into ¼-inch dice (1 cup)

½ medium onion, cut into ¼-inch dice (¾ cup)

4 garlic cloves, minced

1 (24-ounce) jar marinara sauce of your choice (see Tips)

1 teaspoon dried Italian seasoning

1½ cups water

8 ounces gluten-free lasagna noodles, broken into 2-inch pieces

1 cup cottage cheese (or part-skim ricotta)

6 ounces shredded part-skim mozzarella cheese (1½ cups)

Optional toppings:
Chopped fresh basil leaves and/or freshly grated or shaved Parmesan cheese

Tips from the Dietitians
If you're looking to avoid added sugars, use marinara sauce that is made without sugar.

When your to-do list is long and you've got a hungry family to feed, it's tempting to order takeout. But before you grab the phone, consider this skillet lasagna instead. With jumbled-up layers of lean ground beef, curly lasagna noodles, vegetables, and cheese, it's a hearty and wholesome meal the entire family will love—no layering and no fuss required.

Place a 12-inch skillet with a tight-fitting lid over medium-high heat. When hot, add the avocado oil and swirl to coat the bottom. And the beef, zucchini, bell pepper, onion, and garlic. Break up the meat with a wooden spoon and cook, stirring occasionally, until the onion and pepper start to soften and the beef is almost cooked through, 8 to 10 minutes.

Add the marinara sauce, Italian seasoning, and water to the skillet and bring to a boil.

Add the lasagna noodles to the skillet and stir. Decrease the heat to low and cover the skillet with the lid. Cook, stirring every 5 to 7 minutes, until the noodles are tender, 25 to 30 minutes. If the noodles are not fully cooked by this point, add 2 to 4 tablespoons of water and cook, covered, until the noodles are tender.

Uncover and stir in the cottage cheese and half of the mozzarella. Stir and cook, uncovered, for 5 minutes.

Sprinkle the remaining mozzarella over the top of the lasagna. Remove the skillet from the heat, cover, and let the lasagna stand for 5 minutes to allow the sauce to thicken.

If desired, uncover and broil for 3 to 4 minutes to crisp up the mozzarella.

Garnish with chopped fresh basil and serve with Parmesan, if desired.

Store leftovers in an airtight container in the fridge for up to 3 days.

Nutrition Info: (Serving size: ⅛ of the recipe without the optional toppings) 312 calories, 9g total fat, 4g saturated fat, 590mg sodium, 33g carbs, 7g sugar, 3g fiber, 25g protein

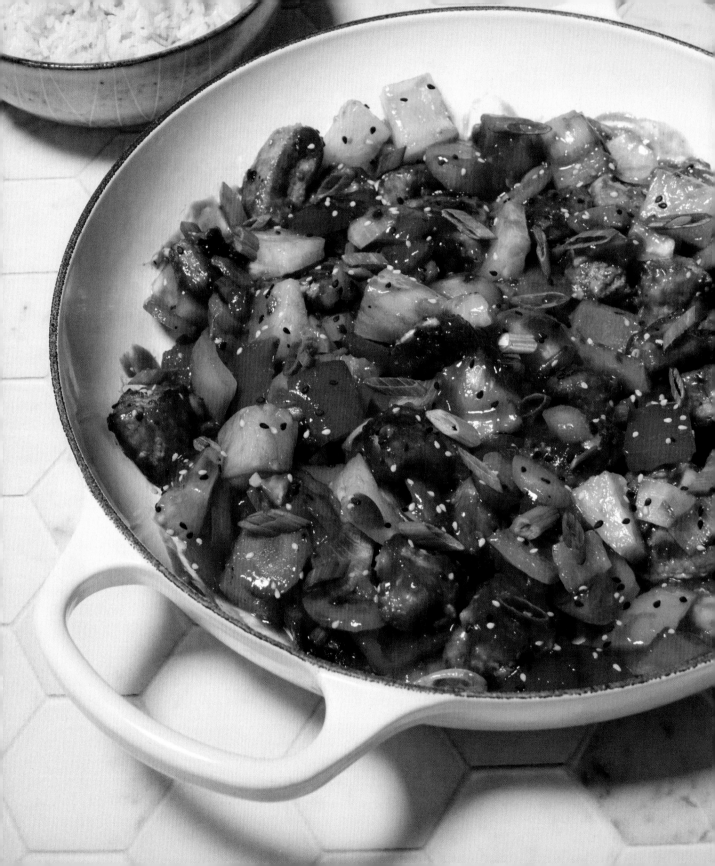

sweet-&-sour pork

Prep Time: **20 minutes** | Cook Time: **20 minutes** | Total Time: **40 minutes** | Makes **4 servings**

1 (14-ounce) can pineapple chunks in juice, drained with ½ cup juice reserved

⅓ cup ketchup (see Tips)

3 tablespoons rice vinegar

2 tablespoons coconut aminos

2 garlic cloves, minced

1 teaspoon grated peeled fresh ginger

1 tablespoon cornstarch (or 1½ tablespoons arrowroot starch, for grain-free)

1 (1-pound) pork tenderloin, trimmed and cut into ¾-inch pieces

½ teaspoon fine salt

⅛ teaspoon ground black pepper

1 tablespoon avocado oil or extra-virgin olive oil, divided

½ medium onion, cut into ¾-inch pieces (1 cup)

2 medium carrots, peeled and thinly sliced on the diagonal (1 cup)

2 medium bell peppers, cut into ¾-inch pieces (any color; 2 cups)

Optional for serving:
Cooked cauliflower rice (for grain-free), Coconut-Lime Rice, or other cooked rice, sesame seeds, and/or thinly sliced green onions

Tips from the Dietitians
If you're looking to avoid added sugars, use ketchup that is made without sugar.

To take out or not to take out? That is often the question in busy households, including our own. Our one-skillet take on a Chinese American restaurant favorite features more vegetables and less sugar. Serve it over cauliflower rice for a lower-carb option or our Coconut-Lime Rice (page 71) for a super kid-friendly meal the whole family will enjoy.

In a small bowl, combine the reserved pineapple juice with the ketchup, vinegar, coconut aminos, garlic, and ginger. Whisk to combine. Slowly whisk in the cornstarch until no lumps remain. Set aside.

In a medium bowl, combine the pork, salt, and pepper. Toss well to coat.

Place a large skillet over medium-high heat. When hot, add 1 teaspoon of the avocado oil and swirl to coat the bottom. When the oil just starts to shimmer, add half of the pork in a single layer and cook, undisturbed, until lightly browned, about 2 minutes. Flip the pork and cook, undisturbed, until lightly browned, about another 2 minutes. Transfer to a plate and repeat with 1 more teaspoon of the oil and the remaining pork. Set the pork aside.

Add the remaining 1 teaspoon oil to the same skillet (no need to wipe it out first) and swirl to coat the bottom. Add the onion and carrots and cook, stirring often, for 4 minutes. Add the bell peppers to the skillet and cook, stirring often, until the vegetables are crisp-tender, about 4 minutes more.

Add the pork and pineapple chunks to the skillet. Stir the sweet-and-sour sauce, then add it to the skillet. Cook, stirring frequently, until the sauce thickens and the vegetables are tender, 5 to 6 minutes.

Remove the skillet from the heat and sprinkle with sesame seeds and/or green onions, if using, and serve with cooked cauliflower rice, if desired.

Store leftovers in an airtight container in the refrigerator for up to 4 days.

Nutrition Info: (Serving size: ¼ of the recipe, about 1¾ cups without rice and the optional toppings) 279 calories, 6g total fat, 1g saturated fat, 719mg sodium, 31g carbs, 18g sugar, 3g fiber, 26g protein

smothered pork chops with mushroom sauce

Prep Time: **15 minutes** | Cook Time: **20 minutes** | Total Time: **35 minutes** | Makes **4 servings**

GF
GrF
DF
EF
NF
NAS

4 bone-in center-cut pork chops (each ¾ to 1 inch thick; about 2 pounds total)
½ teaspoon garlic powder
½ teaspoon onion powder
½ teaspoon fine salt
Ground black pepper
1 tablespoon avocado oil or extra-virgin olive oil, divided
8 ounces button or cremini mushrooms, stemmed and sliced
½ medium yellow onion, sliced (1 cup)
3 garlic cloves, minced
¾ cup low-sodium chicken broth
¾ cup full-fat canned coconut milk
½ teaspoon ground sage
3 cups loosely packed baby spinach (3 ounces)

Tips from the Dietitians

For a thicker sauce, after the spinach has wilted, whisk in 2 teaspoons of thickener, such as cornstarch (or 1 tablespoon arrowroot starch, for grain-free).

Perfectly tender bone-in pork chops are topped with a creamy sauce. We've kept this recipe dairy-free by using coconut milk, but don't you worry, the coconut flavor is very subtle. Serve the pork chops over rice, cauliflower rice, or Instant Pot Garlic Mashed Potatoes (page 62), with a side of Crispy Broccoli (page 70).

Place a large skillet over medium-high heat. While the skillet is heating, sprinkle the pork chops with the garlic powder, onion powder, ¼ teaspoon of the salt, and a dash of black pepper.

When the skillet is hot, add 2 teaspoons of the avocado oil and swirl to coat the bottom. When the oil just starts to shimmer, add the pork chops and cook until lightly browned, 3 to 4 minutes per side. Transfer the pork chops to a plate and cover with an inverted plate to keep warm.

To the same skillet, add the remaining 1 teaspoon oil and swirl to coat the bottom. Add the mushrooms and onion and cook, stirring occasionally, until the onion is translucent and soft, 6 to 7 minutes. Add the garlic and cook, stirring occasionally, for 2 minutes.

Add the broth, coconut milk, sage, the remaining ¼ teaspoon salt, and a dash of pepper to the skillet and stir. Bring to a simmer, then cook until slightly thickened, 4 to 5 minutes.

Return the pork chops to the skillet and cook until the internal temperature of the thickest chop registers 145°F, 3 to 5 minutes. The cooking time will depend on the thickness of the pork chops.

Using tongs, transfer the pork chops to a serving platter and allow to rest while you finish the sauce.

Add the spinach to the sauce in the skillet and cook until wilted, 1 to 2 minutes. Pour the sauce over the pork chops and serve.

Store leftovers in an airtight container in the refrigerator for up to 4 days.

Nutrition Info: (Serving size: 1 pork chop with ⅓ cup sauce) 421 calories, 19g total fat, 10g saturated fat, 486mg sodium, 6g carbs, 3g sugar, 1g fiber, 48g protein

sheet pan pork loin with brussels sprouts & apples

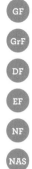

Prep Time: **25 minutes** | Cook Time: **30 minutes** | Total Time: **55 minutes, plus 5 minutes for resting** | Makes **4 servings**

2 tablespoons Dijon mustard

2 tablespoons avocado oil or extra-virgin olive oil, divided

1 tablespoon pure maple syrup (omit for no added sugar)

4 garlic cloves, finely minced

1 tablespoon fresh rosemary, chopped (or 1 teaspoon dried rosemary, lightly crushed)

2 teaspoons fresh thyme leaves (or ¾ teaspoon dried thyme)

¾ teaspoon fine salt

¾ teaspoon ground black pepper

1 (1- to 1¼-pound) boneless pork loin roast, patted dry (see Tips)

1 pound Brussels sprouts, trimmed, and halved if large (4 cups)

2 medium apples (such as Honeycrisp, Braeburn, Pink Lady, or Cripps Pink), cut into ¾-inch chunks

½ medium red onion, sliced ½ inch thick

Tips from the Dietitians

It's best to use a pork loin roast that isn't super thick (about 3 inches in diameter at the thickest point) to get it to cook at the same time as the veggies. But if the pork is done before the vegetables, simply transfer it to a platter and loosely tent with aluminum foil while the vegetables finish cooking.

Weeknight meals don't have to be complicated or involve *every dish in the kitchen* when they're as simple as this one. Everything in this recipe cooks on a single sheet pan. The result is savory, succulent pork loin and tender, flavorful Brussels sprouts and sweet-tart apples. Make this meal and you'll quickly understand why it's a favorite in both of our homes.

Preheat the oven to 400°F. Line a rimmed baking sheet with parchment paper and set aside.

In a small bowl, combine the mustard, 1 tablespoon of the avocado oil, the maple syrup, garlic, rosemary, thyme, ½ teaspoon of the salt, and ½ teaspoon of the pepper and stir.

Place the pork in the center of the baking sheet and rub with the mustard mixture, coating the exposed surface.

Add the Brussels sprouts, apples, and onion to the baking sheet, arranging them around the pork. Drizzle the apples and vegetables with the remaining 1 tablespoon oil, sprinkle with the remaining ¼ teaspoon each salt and pepper, and toss well to coat.

Roast in the oven for 25 to 30 minutes, or until an instant-read thermometer inserted into the thickest part of the pork loin registers 145°F, tossing the apples and vegetables with tongs or a wooden spoon halfway through.

Remove the baking sheet from the oven, tent loosely with aluminum foil, and allow to rest for 5 minutes.

Slice the pork and serve with the apples and vegetables.

Store leftovers in an airtight container in the refrigerator for up to 4 days.

Nutrition Info: (Serving size: ¼ of the recipe) 359 calories, 16g total fat, 4g saturated fat, 535mg sodium, 18g carbs, 16g sugar, 2g fiber, 29g protein

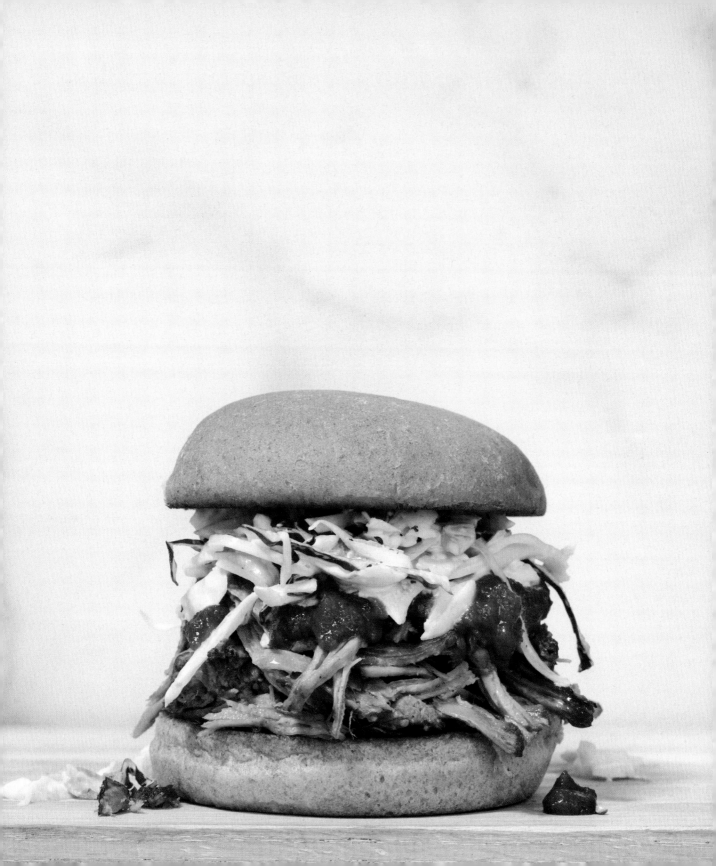

instant pot pulled pork

Prep Time: **15 minutes** | Cook Time: **1 hour 30 minutes** | Total Time: **2 hours 15 minutes, includes 30 minutes for pressure buildup and natural release** | Makes **6 servings**

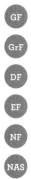

1½ teaspoons garlic powder

1½ teaspoons fine salt

1 teaspoon smoked paprika

1 teaspoon onion powder

½ teaspoon ground black pepper

½ teaspoon chili powder

1 (3-pound) boneless pork shoulder, trimmed of excess fat and patted dry

3 teaspoons avocado oil or extra-virgin olive oil, divided

½ medium onion, thinly sliced (1 cup)

1 cup water

4 garlic cloves, minced

2 teaspoons apple cider vinegar

Whenever we travel together for work we always make a point to find the most popular barbecue joint in town. But when travel isn't on the docket and we don't have time to tend the smoker, we pull out the Instant Pot and let it do the work for us. This crowd-pleasing pulled pork hits the spot, especially when drizzled with our Homemade Barbecue Sauce (page 260) and served alongside our Loaded Baked Potato Salad (page 57), or on a gluten-free bun served alongside a scoop of our Every Occasion Coleslaw (page 59).

In a small bowl, combine the garlic powder, salt, paprika, onion powder, pepper, and chili powder. Rub all over the pork, massaging it into the surface with your fingertips.

Select the sauté function on a 6-quart Instant Pot. When the pot is hot, add 2 teaspoons of the avocado oil. Add the pork and cook 2 minutes per side. Transfer to a plate.

Add the remaining 1 teaspoon oil to the pot immediately followed by the onion and cook, stirring constantly, until the onion is slightly softened and starting to brown on the edges a bit, about 3 minutes. Press cancel on the Instant Pot and add the water. Use a wooden spoon to scrape up any browned bits then stir the garlic into the onions.

Place the pork on top of the onions. Lock the lid in place and switch the valve to the "sealing" position. Set the Instant Pot to cook at high pressure for 90 minutes. (It will take about 10 minutes for the Instant Pot to build up the pressure before the timer starts counting down.)

When the timer goes off, allow the pressure to naturally release for 20 minutes, then switch the vent valve to "venting" to release any residual steam.

Continued on the next page

Transfer the pork to a plate or a shallow dish. Using a slotted spoon, transfer the onion to the dish with the pork, and reserve the cooking liquid. Using two forks, shred the pork into bite-size pieces.

Add 1 to 2 tablespoons of the reserved cooking liquid to the pork, to taste. Add the vinegar and toss to mix well with the pork and onion.

Serve with barbecue sauce and desired sides.

Store leftovers in an airtight container in the refrigerator for up to 4 days or in the freezer for up to 3 months.

Nutrition Info: (Serving size: 4 ounces of pulled pork) 280 calories, 8g total fat, 2g saturated fat, 405mg sodium, 3g carbs, 1g sugar, 0g fiber, 45g protein

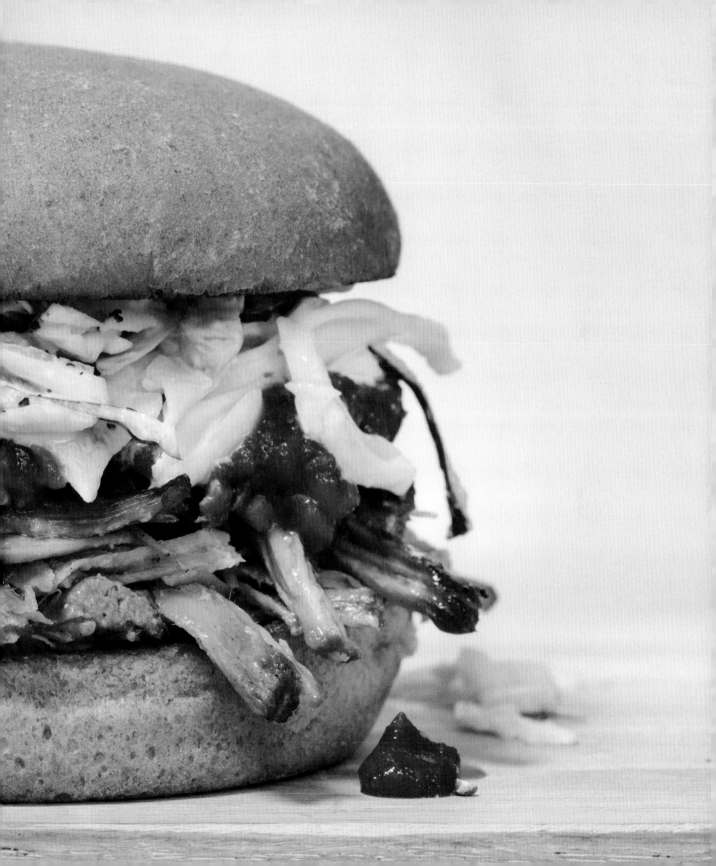

easier-than-ever slow cooker baby back ribs

Prep Time: **20 minutes** | Cook Time: **8 hours 10 minutes** | Total Time: **8 hours 30 minutes** | Makes **4 servings**

GF
GrF
DF
EF
NF
NAS

2½ to 3 pounds pork baby back
    ribs
1 tablespoon light brown sugar
    (omit for no added sugar)
1½ teaspoons garlic powder
1 teaspoon onion powder
1 teaspoon smoked paprika
1 teaspoon chili powder
¾ teaspoon fine salt
½ teaspoon ground black pepper
⅓ cup water
⅔ cup store-bought barbecue
    sauce (or Homemade Barbecue
    Sauce page 260, or see Tips)

If the thought of making barbecued ribs intimidates you, this recipe is for you! Fall-off-the-bone tender ribs can be yours any night of the week, without a grill thanks to our slow cooker method. In fact, they're so easy that the hardest part of the process is deciding which brand of barbecue sauce to use (or use our Homemade Barbecue Sauce). Serve a rack tonight with our Every Occasion Coleslaw (page 59), Ranch Roasted Potatoes (page 61), The Best Broccoli Salad (page 45), or Loaded Baked Potato Salad (page 57), for a meal that delivers big flavors with little effort.

Remove the silver skin (membrane) from the back of the ribs: Slide a butter knife or paring knife under the skin anywhere along each rack of ribs. Use the knife to lift and loosen the skin enough that you can grab it with a paper towel. Pull off and discard the skin. It should come off in one piece. If it doesn't, use the knife to start another section and repeat until you can remove all of it.

Cut the racks into sections of three to four ribs so they will fit in a 6-quart slow cooker.

In a small bowl, combine the brown sugar, garlic powder, onion powder, paprika, chili powder, salt, and pepper and mix to combine. Rub the spice mixture all over the ribs and place them in the slow cooker, overlapping them slightly. Add the water, being careful not to pour it over the seasoned ribs.

Cover the slow cooker and cook on low for 8 hours (or high for 4 hours).

Position the top rack of the oven 6 to 8 inches from the broiler. Preheat the broiler to medium-high.

Transfer the ribs to a baking sheet, arranging them in a single layer, and brush liberally with a third of the barbecue sauce. Broil the ribs for 3 to 4 minutes, or until the sauce starts to bubble and lightly caramelize.

Remove the baking sheet from the oven, flip the ribs, and brush the tops with half of the remaining sauce, reserving the rest for serving. Broil again for 3 to 4 minutes, or until the sauce starts to bubble and lightly caramelize.

Transfer the rib sections to a serving platter (or cut them into individual ribs, if desired) and serve with the remaining barbecue sauce and any of the optional sides.

Store leftovers in an airtight container in the refrigerator for up to 4 days.

Tips from the Dietitians

If you're looking to avoid added sugars, use a barbecue sauce that is made without sugar.

Nutrition Info: (Serving size: ¼ of the recipe without the optional accompaniments) 571 calories, 38g total fat, 13g saturated fat, 780mg sodium, 12g carbs, 9g sugar, 1g fiber, 44g protein

Noodle-Free Veggie Pad Thai with Shrimp

Sheet Pan Fish-&-Chips with Tartar Sauce

Fish Tacos with Avocado "Crema"

Sheet Pan Harissa Salmon with Vegetables

Bruschetta Salmon

Weeknight Salmon Cakes with Lemon-Dill Aioli

Tuna & Egg Salad with Dill

Red Curry Coconut Soup with Shrimp

fish & seafood entrées

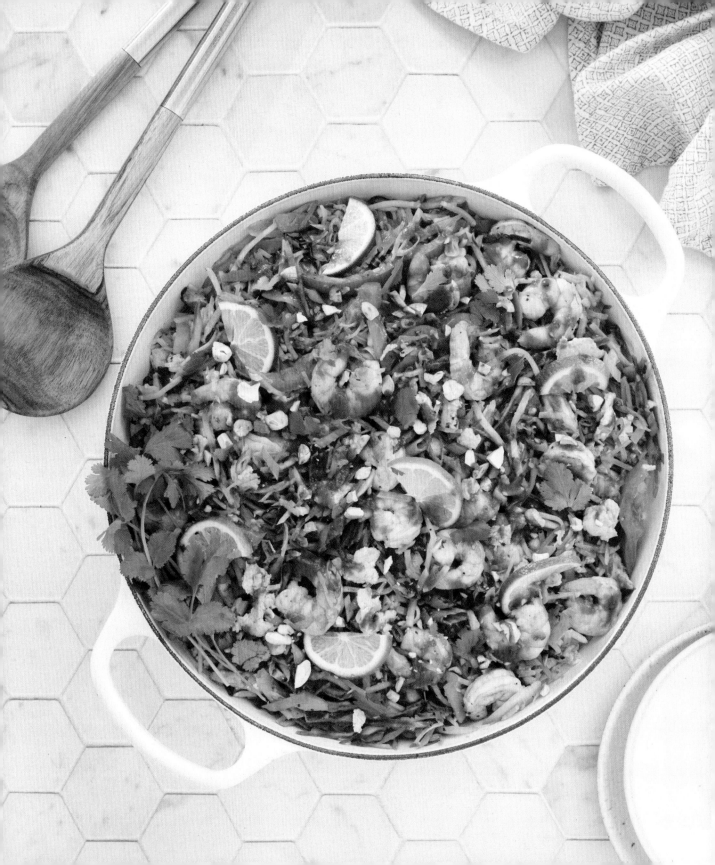

noodle-free veggie pad thai with shrimp

Prep Time: **25 minutes** | Cook Time: **20 minutes** | Total Time: **45 minutes** | Makes **4 servings**

FOR THE SAUCE

¼ cup natural creamy almond butter (or substitute natural creamy peanut butter)

¼ cup coconut aminos

3 tablespoons fresh lime juice (1 medium lime)

2 tablespoons rice vinegar

1 tablespoon toasted sesame oil

½ teaspoon crushed red pepper flakes (optional)

FOR THE SHRIMP AND VEGETABLES

1 pound medium raw shrimp, peeled and deveined, thawed if frozen

1 tablespoon plus 2 teaspoons avocado oil or extra-virgin olive oil, divided

3 large eggs, whisked (omit for egg-free)

Fine salt and ground black pepper

1 (12-ounce) bag broccoli slaw

1½ cups shredded red cabbage

1½ cups shredded peeled carrots

1 medium red bell pepper, sliced (1 cup)

½ medium yellow onion, sliced (1 cup)

4 garlic cloves, minced

2 teaspoons grated peeled fresh ginger (2-inch piece; or substitute ½ teaspoon ground ginger)

6 to 8 green onions, thinly sliced, white/light green and dark green parts separated

¼ cup water

This dish is inspired by one of our favorite take-out meals. Strands of broccoli slaw, shredded cabbage, and carrots stand in for noodles, packing this meal with extra vegetables. The homemade Thai-inspired sauce adds incredible flavor to this one-skillet recipe. We like to chop and shred the vegetables a day or two before it's on the menu, for a fast and easy weeknight meal.

Make the sauce: Combine the almond butter, coconut aminos, lime juice, vinegar, sesame oil, and pepper flakes, if using, in a small bowl and whisk until well combined and smooth.

Prepare the shrimp: Place the shrimp in a colander and rinse under cold water. Drain, then transfer to a plate, pat dry with paper towels, and set aside.

For the vegetables: Place a large skillet (at least 12 inches) over medium heat. When hot, add the 2 teaspoons avocado oil and swirl to coat the bottom. Add the eggs, season with salt and black pepper, and cook, stirring often with a rubber spatula to scramble the eggs, until set, 2 to 4 minutes. Transfer to a plate and set aside. Wipe the skillet clean and return it to the stove.

To the same skillet over medium heat, add the remaining 1 tablespoon oil and swirl to coat the bottom. Add the broccoli slaw, cabbage, carrots, bell pepper, onion, garlic, ginger, and white/light green parts of the green onion, along with the water. Season with salt and pepper. Cook, tossing often, until the vegetables are partially cooked through, 7 to 8 minutes.

Push the vegetables to one side of the skillet and add the shrimp to the other side. Cook, tossing the shrimp occasionally, until the shrimp is almost cooked through, about 4 minutes. Using tongs, combine the shrimp and vegetables and continue to cook, tossing occasionally, until the vegetables are tender.

Continued on the next page

Optional toppings:
Chopped fresh cilantro leaves, roughly chopped dry-roasted cashews, toasted sesame seeds, sliced green onions, and/or lime wedges

Add the sauce and dark green parts of the green onion. Using tongs, carefully toss all the ingredients to combine and cook until heated through, 1 to 2 minutes. Top with the scrambled eggs and stir in gently.

Serve with your desired toppings. Add salt and pepper to taste.

Store leftovers in an airtight container in the refrigerator for up to 3 days.

Nutrition Info: (Serving size: 2 heaping cups without the optional toppings) 469 calories, 27g total fat, 4g saturated fat, 699mg sodium, 27g carbs, 15g sugar, 5g fiber, 33g protein

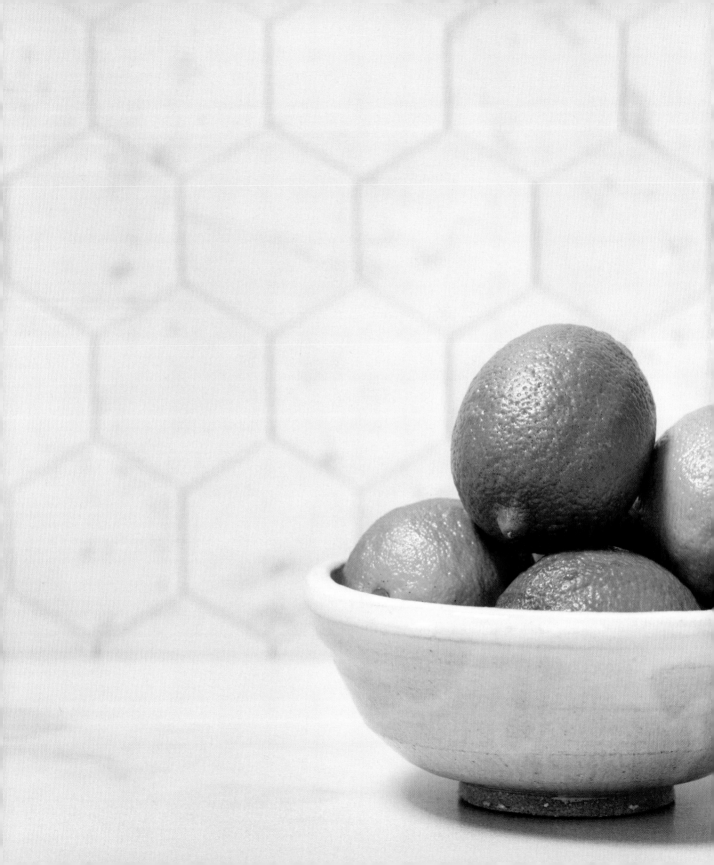

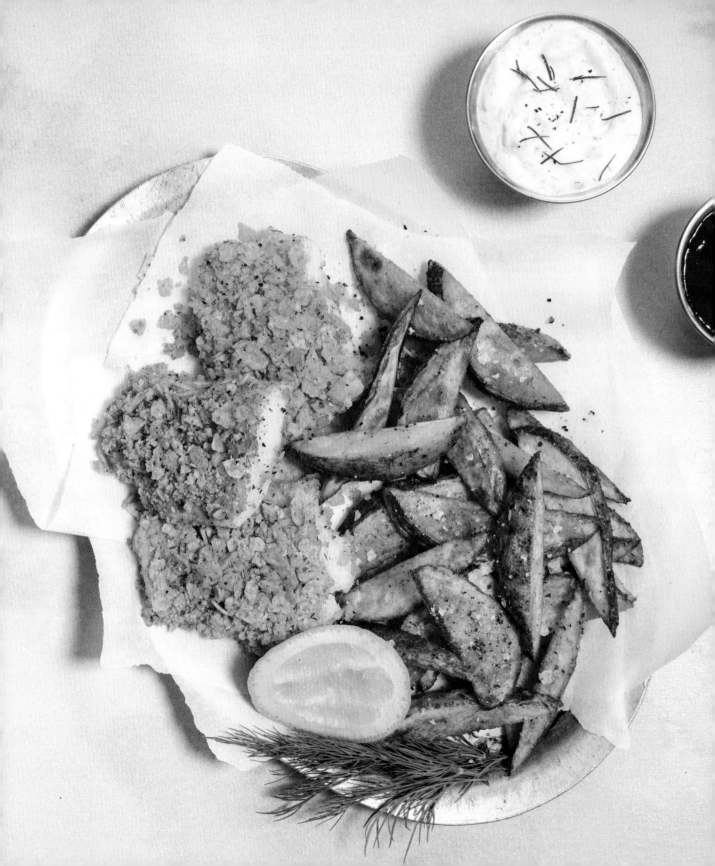

sheet pan fish-&-chips with tartar sauce

Prep Time: **20 minutes** | Cook Time: **30 minutes** | Total Time: **50 minutes** | Makes **4 servings**

FOR THE TARTAR SAUCE

⅓ cup mayonnaise (see Tips)
2 tablespoons pickle relish or chopped dill pickles
¼ teaspoon dried dill
Fine salt (optional)

FOR THE CHIPS

3 medium russet potatoes (1¼ pounds), scrubbed clean and cut into ¼-inch wedges
1 tablespoon avocado oil or extra-virgin olive oil
½ teaspoon garlic powder
¼ teaspoon paprika
¼ teaspoon fine salt

FOR THE FISH

3 ounces tortilla chips, crushed to make 1 cup crumbs
1½ teaspoons garlic powder
½ teaspoon onion powder
¼ teaspoon paprika
¼ teaspoon dried thyme
¼ teaspoon fine salt
¼ teaspoon ground black pepper
1 pound cod fillets, about 1 inch thick, cut into 8 equal pieces
1 tablespoon avocado oil or extra-virgin olive oil
Nonstick cooking spray
Lemon wedges, for serving

Tips from the Dietitians

Use vegan mayonnaise to make the tartar sauce egg-free.

We lightened up a pub food favorite by swapping out the beer batter and deep-fat fryer for crushed tortilla chips and the oven. Our version of fish-and-chips keeps all of the flavors and crunch of the real deal while turning it into a healthy weeknight meal your family will love.

Preheat the oven to 425°F. Line a baking sheet with parchment paper.

Make the tartar sauce: In a small bowl, combine the mayo, pickle relish, and dill, and stir. Taste and add salt, if desired. Refrigerate until ready to serve.

Make the chips: In a large bowl, combine the potato wedges with the avocado oil, garlic powder, paprika, and salt, and toss. Transfer the potatoes to the prepared baking sheet and spread them into a single layer. Bake for 20 minutes, flipping the potatoes halfway through.

Meanwhile, make the fish: In a shallow dish, combine the chip crumbs with the garlic powder, onion powder, paprika, thyme, salt, and pepper.

Place the fish on a plate and pat dry with a paper towel. Drizzle the fish with the avocado oil, then carefully roll each piece in the seasoned crumbs until well coated, pressing to help the crumbs adhere.

After the potatoes have baked for 20 minutes, remove the baking sheet from the oven and push the potatoes to one side. Add the fish in a single layer to the other side of the baking sheet and lightly spray each piece with cooking spray. Bake for about 10 minutes, or until the fish flakes easily with a fork.

Transfer the fish-and-chips to a serving platter and serve with the tartar sauce and lemon wedges.

Store leftovers in an airtight container in the refrigerator for up to 3 days.

Nutrition Info: (Serving size: 2 pieces fish plus ¼ of the potatoes plus 2 tablespoons tartar sauce) 475 calories, 22g total fat, 3g saturated fat, 723mg sodium, 45g carbs, 4g sugar, 6g fiber, 26g protein

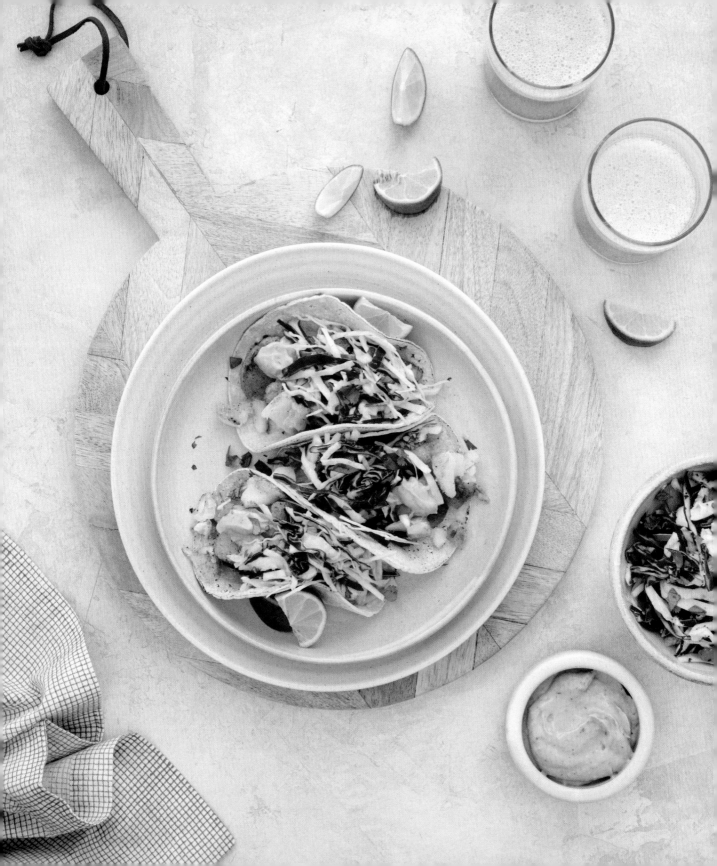

fish tacos with avocado "crema"

Prep Time: **20 minutes** | Cook Time: **10 minutes** | Total Time: **30 minutes** | Makes **4 servings**

GF
DF
EF
NF
NAS

FOR THE AVOCADO "CREMA"

1 medium avocado, peeled or
  scooped from the skin
¼ cup loosely packed fresh
  cilantro leaves, roughly
  chopped
1 garlic clove, minced
3 tablespoons fresh lime juice
  (1 medium lime)
¼ teaspoon fine salt

FOR THE TACOS

½ cup gluten-free all-purpose
  flour blend
¾ teaspoon chili powder
½ teaspoon ground cumin
½ teaspoon garlic powder
¼ teaspoon onion powder
¾ teaspoon fine salt
¼ teaspoon ground black pepper
1 pound cod fillets, patted dry
  and cut crosswise into 8 pieces,
  each about ½ inch wide
2 tablespoons avocado oil or
  extra-virgin olive oil, divided
8 corn tortillas
2⅔ cups Cilantro-Lime Slaw

Optional for serving:
Chopped fresh cilantro leaves
  and/or lime wedges

Jessica's obsession with fish tacos started while living in Alaska during her dietetic internship. These tacos are a healthier version of one of her favorite comfort foods. Instead of the usual deep-frying, hunks of white fish are panfried, then topped with a dairy-free avocado-based "crema" and Cilantro-Lime Slaw (page 58).

Make the avocado "crema": In a food processor, combine the avocado, cilantro, garlic, lime juice, and salt. Process until smooth and the consistency of a thick salad dressing, adding 2 to 3 tablespoons water, if necessary. Set aside.

Make the tacos: In a shallow dish, combine the flour, chili powder, cumin, garlic powder, onion powder, salt, and pepper. Mix with a fork to combine.

Carefully roll each piece of fish in the seasoned flour to coat all sides.

Place a large skillet over medium-high heat. When hot, add 1 tablespoon of the avocado oil and swirl to coat the bottom. When the oil is hot, add 4 pieces of the fish and cook until ready to flip, about 3 minutes. The fish is ready to flip when the underside is golden brown and releases easily from the skillet. Flip each piece with a spatula and cook until the fish flakes easily with a fork, 2 to 3 minutes, keeping in mind that the cooking time will depend on the thickness of the fish. Transfer the cooked fish to a plate and repeat with the remaining 1 tablespoon oil and 4 pieces fish.

To warm the tortillas, place another large skillet over medium-high heat. When hot, add 1 to 2 tortillas and cook 30 seconds per side. Transfer to a plate and cover with a clean kitchen towel to keep them warm. Repeat with the remaining tortillas.

Serve the fish with the warm corn tortillas, Avocado "Crema," and Cilantro-Lime Slaw. Store leftovers in separate airtight containers in the refrigerator for up to 3 days.

Nutrition Info: (Serving size: 2 tacos plus 3 tablespoons crema plus ⅔ cup slaw) 419 calories, 14g total fat, 1g saturated fat, 865mg sodium, 45g carbs, 5g sugar, 8g fiber, 27g protein

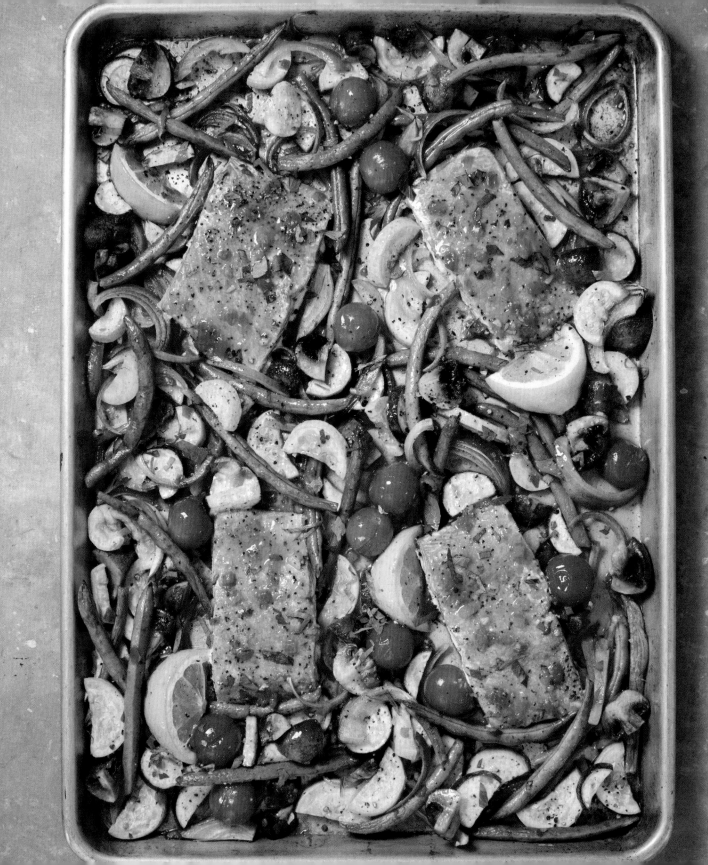

sheet pan harissa salmon with vegetables

Prep Time: **20 minutes** | Cook Time: **25 minutes** | Total Time: **45 minutes** | Makes **4 servings**

GF
GrF
DF
EF
NF
NAS

4 skin-on salmon fillets (1 to 1¼ pounds)

Fine salt and ground black pepper

2 small zucchini and/or yellow summer squash, sliced into ¼-inch-thick half-moons

12 ounces fresh green beans, trimmed (2 cups)

8 ounces cremini mushrooms, stemmed and quartered (3 cups)

6 ounces grape tomatoes (1 cup)

½ medium red onion, thinly sliced (1 cup)

3 tablespoons harissa sauce (mild or spicy; we use the Mina brand)

2 tablespoons avocado oil or extra-virgin olive oil

3 garlic cloves, minced

2 lemons, 1 juiced (3 to 4 tablespoons) and the other cut into 4 wedges

Optional for garnish:
Chopped fresh parsley

Sheet pan meals make busy weeknights a whole lot easier by cutting down on cleanup time. Here we combine tender fillets of heart-healthy salmon with a rainbow of vegetables on a single baking sheet. We season both the fish and the vegetables with harissa, a spicy and aromatic condiment made of chiles, citrus, spices, and oil that is a staple in North African and Middle Eastern dishes.

Preheat the oven to 425°F. Line a rimmed baking sheet with parchment paper and set aside.

Place the salmon, skin side down, on a plate. Sprinkle with ¼ teaspoon salt and a pinch of pepper and set aside.

Spread the squash, green beans, mushrooms, tomatoes, and onion on the prepared baking sheet.

In a small bowl, whisk the harissa, avocado oil, garlic, and lemon juice. Pour all but 2 tablespoons of the harissa mixture over the vegetables on the baking sheet and toss to coat; spread the vegetables into a single layer. Add the lemon wedges to the baking sheet.

Roast the vegetables in the oven for about 12 minutes, or until they start to soften. Remove from the oven and make room for the salmon.

Add the salmon, skin side down, and spread the remaining 2 tablespoons harissa mixture onto the fillets. Roast for 8 to 12 minutes, or until the salmon flakes easily with a fork.

Remove the baking sheet from the oven. Add salt and pepper to taste and garnish with parsley, if using. Serve the salmon and vegetables with the roasted lemon wedges.

Store leftovers in an airtight container in the refrigerator for up to 4 days.

Nutrition Info: (Serving size: 1 fillet plus ¼ of the veggies) 354 calories, 19g total fat, 5g saturated fat, 402mg sodium, 16g carbs, 8g sugar, 5g fiber, 31g protein

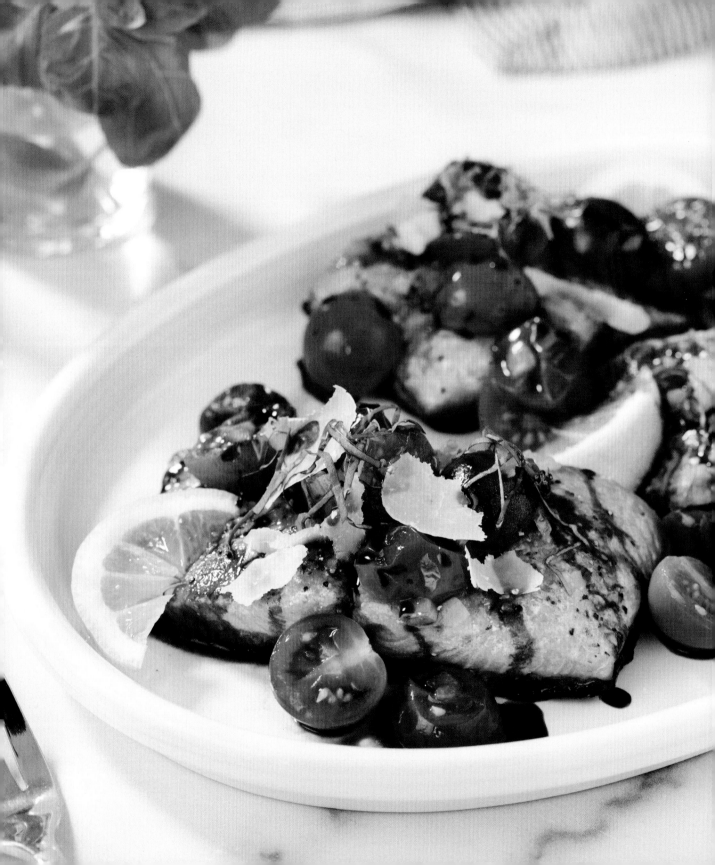

bruschetta salmon

Prep Time: **15 minutes** | Cook Time: **25 minutes** | Total Time: **40 minutes** | Makes **4 servings**

GF

GrF

DFO

EF

NF

NAS

⅔ cup balsamic vinegar

4 teaspoons avocado oil or extra-virgin olive oil, divided

4 (5-ounce) skin-on salmon fillets, patted dry and kept at room temperature for 20 minutes

Fine salt and ground black pepper

1 medium shallot, finely diced (⅓ cup)

1 pint grape tomatoes, halved (2 cups)

3 garlic cloves, minced

1 lemon, half juiced, the remaining half cut into quarters for serving

¼ cup chopped or sliced fresh basil leaves

¼ cup freshly grated or shaved Parmesan cheese (omit for dairy-free)

We took one of our favorite appetizers and paired it with heart-healthy, protein-rich salmon to create a main dish that's worthy of serving at a dinner party. The balsamic glaze is simple to make and takes the dish from really good to lick-the-plate-clean good.

Place a small saucepan over medium heat. Add the balsamic vinegar and bring it just to a boil. Decrease the heat and simmer until reduced by half and the balsamic glaze is glossy and thick enough to coat a spoon, 10 to 12 minutes. Remove from the heat and allow to cool. The glaze will thicken a bit more as it cools.

While the balsamic glaze simmers, place a large skillet over medium-high heat. When the skillet is hot, add 2 teaspoons of the avocado oil and swirl to coat the bottom. Add the salmon fillets skin side down, season with salt and pepper, and cook, undisturbed, for 10 minutes. Cover the skillet partially and cook, undisturbed, until the salmon flakes easily with a fork, 3 to 5 minutes. Remove the salmon to a platter and set aside.

Add the remaining 2 teaspoons oil to the skillet and swirl to coat the bottom. Add the shallot and cook, stirring constantly, for about 3 minutes, or until the shallot is transluscent. Add the tomatoes and garlic to the skillet. Season with salt and pepper and continue to cook, stirring occasionally, just until the tomatoes start to soften, 4 to 5 minutes. Stir in the lemon juice and remove the skillet from the heat.

Spoon the tomato mixture over the salmon fillets. Drizzle with 2 tablespoons of the balsamic glaze, sprinkle with the basil and Parmesan, and serve with the lemon wedges.

Store leftover salmon and vegetables in an airtight container in the refrigerator for up to 3 days. Store any leftover balsamic glaze in an airtight container in the refrigerator for up to 2 weeks.

Nutrition Info: (Serving size: ¼ of the recipe) 379 calories, 17g total fat, 3g saturated fat, 225mg sodium, 19g carbs, 17g sugar, 0g fiber, 35g protein

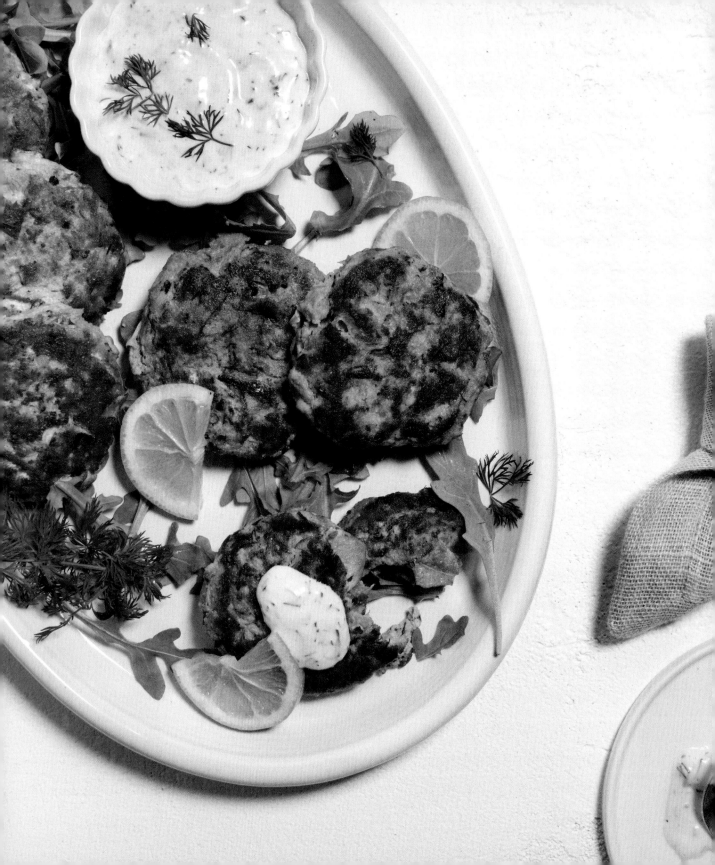

weeknight salmon cakes with lemon-dill aioli

Prep Time: **15 minutes** | Cook Time: **10 minutes** | Total Time: **25 minutes** | Makes **4 servings**

GF
GrF
DF
NFO
NAS

FOR THE SALMON CAKES

12 ounces skin-on salmon fillets
  (2 to 3 fillets)
1 tablespoon plus 2 teaspoons
  avocado oil or extra-virgin olive
  oil
Fine salt and ground black pepper
2 large eggs
¼ cup almond flour (or substitute
  gluten-free bread crumbs)
2 tablespoons fresh lemon juice
  (½ lemon)
2 green onions, white and light
  green parts only, roughly
  chopped (2 to 3 tablespoons)
1 tablespoon chopped fresh dill
2 teaspoons Dijon mustard
1 teaspoon garlic powder

FOR THE LEMON-DILL AIOLI

¼ cup mayonnaise (see Tips)
1 tablespoon chopped fresh dill,
  plus more for garnish (optional)
1½ teaspoons fresh lemon juice
1 teaspoon Dijon mustard
¼ teaspoon finely grated lemon
  zest
Fine salt and ground black pepper

Tips from the Dietitians

Make sure that the skillet and
the oil are hot before adding the
salmon cakes.

If you're looking to avoid added
sugars, use mayonnaise that is
made without sugar.

These easy salmon cakes are a great way to sneak more healthy fats into your diet, and when topped with creamy lemon-dill aioli, they're anything but ordinary!

Start the salmon cakes: Preheat the oven to 425°F. Line a rimmed baking sheet with parchment paper.

Place the salmon, skin side down, on the baking sheet. Brush ½ teaspoon of the avocado oil over each fillet and season with salt and pepper.

Bake for 8 to 12 minutes, or until the salmon flakes easily with a fork. Remove the baking sheet from the oven and let the salmon rest until cool enough to handle, 5 to 10 minutes. Remove and discard the skin, then use your hands to break up the salmon into small pieces.

While the salmon is in the oven, make the Lemon-Dill Aioli: In a small bowl, combine the mayonnaise, dill, lemon juice, mustard, and lemon zest and stir to mix well. Add salt and pepper to taste. Garnish with additional dill, if desired. Refrigerate until ready to serve.

Form and cook the salmon cakes: In a medium bowl, combine the salmon, eggs, almond flour, lemon juice, green onions, dill, mustard, garlic powder, ¼ teaspoon salt, and ¼ teaspoon pepper and mix well. Form into 8 small patties. Handle carefully—the patties fall apart easily until they are cooked.

Place a skillet over medium-high heat. Add the remaining 1 tablespoon oil and swirl to coat the bottom. Once the oil is hot, carefully add the patties and cook for 5 minutes. Slide a spatula underneath 1 patty at a time to carefully flip and cook until cooked through, 4 to 5 minutes. To serve, top the salmon cakes with 1 to 2 tablespoons of the aioli.

Store leftovers in separate airtight containers in the refrigerator for up to 4 days or store the salmon cakes in the freezer for up to 3 months.

Nutrition Info: (Serving size: 2 cakes with 1½ tablespoons of the aioli), 316 calories, 24g total fat, 4g saturated fat, 703mg sodium, 3g carbs, 1g sugar, 1g fiber, 22g protein

tuna & egg salad with dill

Prep Time: **15 minutes** | Total Time: **15 minutes** | Makes **4 servings**

GF
GrF
DF
EFO
NF
NAS

2 (5-ounce) cans water-packed
   tuna, drained
2 Easy-Peel Hard-Boiled Eggs,
   diced (omit for egg-free)
¼ cup finely diced celery
1 to 2 dill pickles, diced (about
   ¼ cup)
3 tablespoons finely diced red
   onion
⅓ cup mayonnaise (or vegan
   mayonnaise, for egg-free; see
   Tips)
2 tablespoons fresh lemon juice
   (½ medium lemon)
1 teaspoon Dijon mustard
1 teaspoon fresh dill, chopped or
   ¼ teaspoon dried dill
¼ teaspoon garlic powder
Fine salt and ground black pepper

Optional for serving:
Butter lettuce or green leaf
   lettuce leaves, vegetable sticks
   and slices, gluten-free tortillas,
   sandwich bread, or crackers

This tuna salad is the real "dill," people! Our twist on the classic corner deli tuna salad includes dill for a bright flavor and chopped Easy-Peel Hard-Boiled Eggs (page 211) for great texture. (The egg yolks also provide choline, which supports a variety of functions in the body, including metabolism.) Tuna salad isn't only for lunch. Enjoy it as a protein-packed snack with fresh vegetables and/or crackers for scooping it up.

In a medium bowl, combine the tuna, eggs, celery, pickles, and onion. Set aside.

In a small bowl, combine the mayonnaise, lemon juice, mustard, dill, garlic powder, and a pinch of pepper and stir to mix well. Pour over the tuna mixture and mix until well combined. Add salt to taste.

Serve the tuna salad tucked in butter lettuce or green leaf lettuce leaves or tortillas, with vegetable sticks and slices, between sandwich bread, or on top of crackers, if desired.

Store leftovers in an airtight container in the refrigerator for up to 3 days.

Tips from the Dietitians
For a creamier tuna salad, add 1 to 2 more tablespoons of mayonnaise to the dressing. If you're looking to avoid added sugars, use mayonnaise that is made without sugar.

Nutrition Info: (Serving size: heaping ½ cup without the optional accompaniments) 234 calories, 17g total fat, 3g saturated fat, 587mg sodium, 2g carbs, 1g sugar, 1g fiber, 17g protein

red curry coconut soup with shrimp

Prep Time: **15 minutes** | Cook Time: **30 minutes** | Total Time: **45 minutes** | Makes **4 servings**

GF
GrF
DF
EF
NF
NAS

2 teaspoons avocado oil or extra-virgin olive oil
1 medium red bell pepper, thinly sliced (1cup)
3 green onions, thinly sliced, white/light green and dark green parts separated
2 garlic cloves, minced
1 teaspoon grated peeled fresh ginger
1 teaspoon grated lime zest
4 cups low-sodium chicken broth
8 ounces shiitake mushrooms (or substitute cremini or button mushrooms), rough stems removed, sliced (2 cups)
1½ tablespoons Thai red curry paste
1 pound medium raw shrimp, peeled and deveined, thawed if frozen
1 (14-ounce) can full-fat coconut milk
2 teaspoons fish sauce
2 tablespoons fresh lime juice (1 medium lime)
2 cups loosely packed baby spinach
½ cup loosely packed fresh cilantro leaves, roughly chopped
Lime wedges, for serving (optional)

Tips from the Dietitians
This soup is particularly delicious when served with a scoop of steamed jasmine rice or our Coconut-Lime Rice (page 71).

While not authentic, this is definitely a delicious and approachable nod to tom kha, which we adapted into a flavorful soup for all to enjoy. We substitute lime zest and ginger for the lemongrass and galangal called for in the traditional Thai version, which helps make this recipe more accessible to everyone.

Place a medium saucepan over medium-high heat. When hot, add the avocado oil and swirl to coat the bottom. Add the bell pepper and the white and light green parts of the green onions. Cook, stirring occasionally, until the pepper just begins to soften, about 4 minutes.

Add the garlic, ginger, and lime zest and continue to cook, stirring, until fragrant, about 1 minute. Add the chicken broth, mushrooms, and curry paste. Increase the heat and bring the soup just to a boil. Decrease the heat enough to maintain a gentle simmer. Simmer, uncovered, for 15 minutes.

Meanwhile, prepare the shrimp: Place the shrimp in a colander and rinse under cold water. Drain, then transfer to a plate, pat dry with paper towels, and set aside.

Add the coconut milk and shrimp to the saucepan, stir, and cook until the shrimp is pink and cooked through, 5 to 7 minutes.

Remove the saucepan from the heat and stir in the fish sauce, lime juice, spinach, cilantro, and dark green parts of the green onion. Allow the spinach a minute or two to wilt before serving.

Serve the soup with lime wedges, if desired.

Store leftovers in an airtight container in the refrigerator for up to 4 days or store in the freezer for up to 3 months.

Nutrition Info: (Serving size: 2 cups) 354 calories, 19g total fat, 16g saturated fat, 799mg sodium, 14g carbs, 5g sugar, 3g fiber, 30g protein

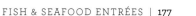

meatless entrées & more

Minestrone Soup

Curried Lentil Stew with Sweet Potatoes & Cauliflower

Rainbow Quinoa Bowls with Peanut Dressing

Spaghetti Squash Pasta & Broccoli with Dairy-Free Alfredo

Sweet Potato & Black Bean Burrito Bowls

Dairy-Free Mac & "Cheese"

Mediterranean Pasta Salad

Oven-Roasted Tomato Soup

Warm Butternut Squash & Kale Salad

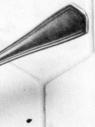

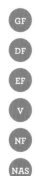

minestrone soup

Prep Time: **20 minutes** | Cook Time: **55 minutes** | Total Time: **1 hour 15 minutes** | Makes **6 servings**

2 tablespoons avocado oil or extra-virgin olive oil

1 medium onion, diced (1½ cups)

7 garlic cloves, minced

2 celery ribs, diced (¾ cup)

2 medium carrots, peeled and diced (1 cup)

8 ounces cremini or button mushrooms, stemmed and sliced (2 to 2½ cups)

4 cups low-sodium vegetable broth or water

1 (28-ounce) can crushed tomatoes

1 (14-ounce) can red kidney beans, drained and rinsed

1 medium zucchini, diced (1½ cups)

1 tablespoon dried Italian seasoning

¾ teaspoon fine salt, plus more as needed

¼ teaspoon ground black pepper, plus more as needed

4 ounces uncooked gluten-free pasta of choice, such as elbows or small shells

Optional for serving:

Chopped fresh parsley and/ or freshly grated or shaved Parmesan cheese (omit for dairy-free and vegan)

If you're looking for a plant-based bowl of soup that you can really tuck into when the weather turns cold, this is the one. It's cozy and hearty thanks to a rich tomato-infused broth, a variety of vegetables, and fiber-rich beans. The soup can be served alongside your favorite sandwich or salad, but can also be a meal on its own with a hunk of crusty bread. We think that it's particularly wonderful topped with grated or shaved Parmesan cheese (but feel free to omit it to keep the dish vegan). Snowstorm optional.

Place a large saucepan or Dutch oven over medium heat. When hot, add the avocado oil and swirl to coat the bottom. Add the onion, garlic, celery, carrots, and mushrooms and cook, stirring occasionally, until the vegetables start to soften, about 8 minutes.

Add the broth, tomatoes, beans, zucchini, Italian seasoning, salt, and pepper to the saucepan and stir. Increase the heat to high and bring just to a boil. Decrease the heat to low. Cover and cook, adjusting the heat as needed to maintain a steady simmer, until the carrots and celery are tender, 40 to 45 minutes.

While the soup simmers, bring a medium pot of salted water to a boil. Cook the pasta according to the package directions. Drain and set aside.

Remove the soup from the heat and stir in the parsley, if using. Add more salt and pepper to taste.

To serve, place a serving of pasta in each bowl and ladle the soup over the pasta. Top with Parmesan, if using.

Store leftovers in separate airtight containers in the refrigerator for up to 4 days.

Tips from the Dietitians

If you plan to have leftovers, refrigerate the pasta and soup separately, then reheat them together in a pot before serving.

Nutrition Info: (Serving size: 2 cups soup plus ½ cup cooked pasta, without the optional ingredients) 215 calories, 5g total fat, 1g saturated fat, 421mg sodium, 34g carbs, 9g sugar, 11g fiber, 9g protein

curried lentil stew with sweet potatoes & cauliflower

Prep Time: **20 minutes** | Cook Time: **30 minutes** | Total Time: **50 minutes** | Makes **6 servings**

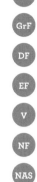

2 teaspoons avocado oil or extra-virgin olive oil

½ medium yellow onion, diced

4 garlic cloves, minced

3 tablespoons curry powder, plus more as needed

1½ teaspoons ground ginger

1 cup red lentils, rinsed and drained

4 cups low-sodium vegetable broth, divided

1 medium to large sweet potato (10 to 12 ounces), peeled and cut into ½-inch cubes

3 cups bite-size cauliflower florets or 1 (10-ounce) bag raw cauliflower florets

1 medium red bell pepper, diced (about 1 cup)

1 small zucchini, halved or quartered lengthwise then sliced crosswise ½ inch thick (1 cup)

1 bunch curly kale, ribs removed and leaves chopped (4 cups)

1 (14-ounce) can full-fat coconut milk

1 teaspoon fine salt, plus more as needed

¼ teaspoon ground black pepper, plus more as needed

Optional toppings:
Chopped fresh basil or cilantro leaves, chopped roasted cashews, and/or lime wedges

This stew is inspired by a red lentil dish that we enjoyed at an Indian restaurant while in San Francisco for a work trip. We added cauliflower, bell pepper, zucchini, and kale to create a veggie-filled one-bowl meal. The curry powder gives it a little kick, while the rich coconut milk–based broth and sweet potatoes lend it just the right amount of natural sweetness. While delicious on its own, the stew pairs well with steamed rice or Coconut-Lime Rice (page 71), or a side of crusty bread. It's guaranteed to warm you from the inside out.

Place a medium saucepan or Dutch oven over medium-high heat. When hot, add the avocado oil and swirl to coat the bottom. Add the onion, garlic, curry powder, and ginger. Cook, stirring occasionally, until the onion is fragrant and translucent, 3 to 4 minutes.

Add the lentils and 2 cups of the broth to the saucepan. Bring to a boil, then decrease the heat to low, cover, and cook until the lentils are partially cooked, about 10 minutes. Adjust the heat as needed to maintain a steady simmer,

To the saucepan, add the sweet potato, cauliflower, bell pepper, zucchini, and the remaining 2 cups broth and stir. Bring to a gentle simmer, cover, and cook until the sweet potato is tender, 10 to 12 minutes.

Stir in the kale, coconut milk, salt, and black pepper. Cook, uncovered, until heated through and the kale is wilted, about 5 minutes. Taste, and add more curry powder, salt, and black pepper, if needed.

Serve the stew with your desired toppings.

Store leftovers in an airtight container in the refrigerator for up to 4 days or in the freezer for up to 3 months.

Nutrition Info: (Serving size: 1½ cups without rice and the optional toppings) 279 calories, 13g total fat, 10g saturated fat, 683mg sodium, 31g carbs, 9g sugar, 10g fiber, 10g protein

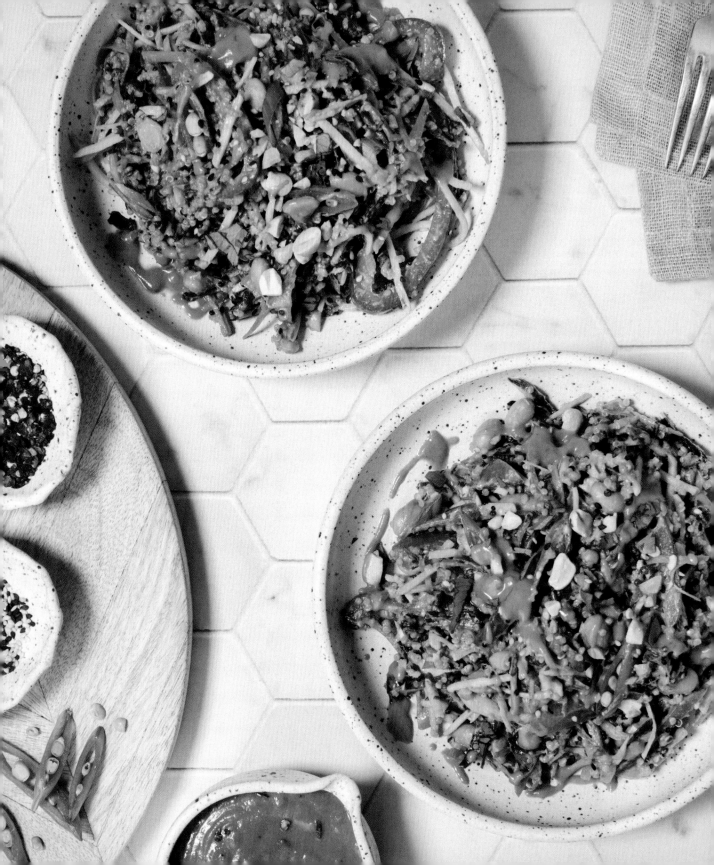

rainbow quinoa bowls with peanut dressing

Prep Time: **30 minutes** | Cook Time: **15 minutes** | Total Time: **45 minutes** | Makes **4 servings**

GF DF EF V NAS NFO

FOR THE SALAD

½ cup uncooked quinoa

1 cup water

2 cups shredded cabbage (any color)

1 cup shredded carrots

1 cup broccoli slaw (or substitute additional cabbage or carrots)

1 cup sliced sugar snap peas

1 cup shelled edamame (see Tips), cooked according to the package directions

1 red bell pepper, thinly sliced (1 cup)

½ cup loosely packed fresh cilantro leaves, roughly chopped

½ cup salted dry-roasted peanuts, roughly chopped (see Tips)

6 green onions, trimmed and thinly sliced (⅓ cup)

2 teaspoons sesame seeds

Peanut Dressing and Dipping Sauce (page 261; see Tips)

Optional toppings:

Roughly chopped roasted peanuts (see Tips), chopped fresh cilantro leaves, and/or lime wedges

This salad packs a plant-based protein punch thanks to quinoa and edamame. We love it because not only is it hearty and satisfying, it's loaded with antioxidants from cabbage, bell peppers, carrots, and sugar snap peas. It's basically a rainbow in a bowl.

Make the salad: Rinse the quinoa in a fine-mesh strainer under cool running water for 30 seconds. Transfer to a small saucepan, add the water, and bring to a boil over medium heat. Decrease the heat to medium low and simmer until all of the water is absorbed, 12 to 15 minutes.

Remove the saucepan from the heat, cover, and let stand for 5 to 10 minutes. Uncover and fluff the quinoa with a fork and set aside to cool.

In a large bowl, combine the cabbage, carrots, broccoli slaw, sugar snap peas, edamame, bell pepper, cilantro, peanuts, green onions, sesame seeds, and cooled quinoa.

Pour the dressing over the salad and toss gently to combine.

To serve, top with chopped peanuts, chopped cilantro, and a squeeze of lime juice, if desired.

Store leftovers in an airtight container in the refrigerator for up to 4 days.

Tips from the Dietitians

Look for shelled edamame in the freezer section.

To make this recipe peanut-free, use almond or cashew butter in the dressing and almonds or cashews for topping.

For a nut-free option, use sunflower seed butter and sunflower or pumpkin seeds for topping.

Nutrition Info: (Serving size: 1½ cups without additional toppings) 430 calories, 23g total fat, 4g saturated fat, 608mg sodium, 43g carbs, 14g sugar, 10g fiber, 19g protein

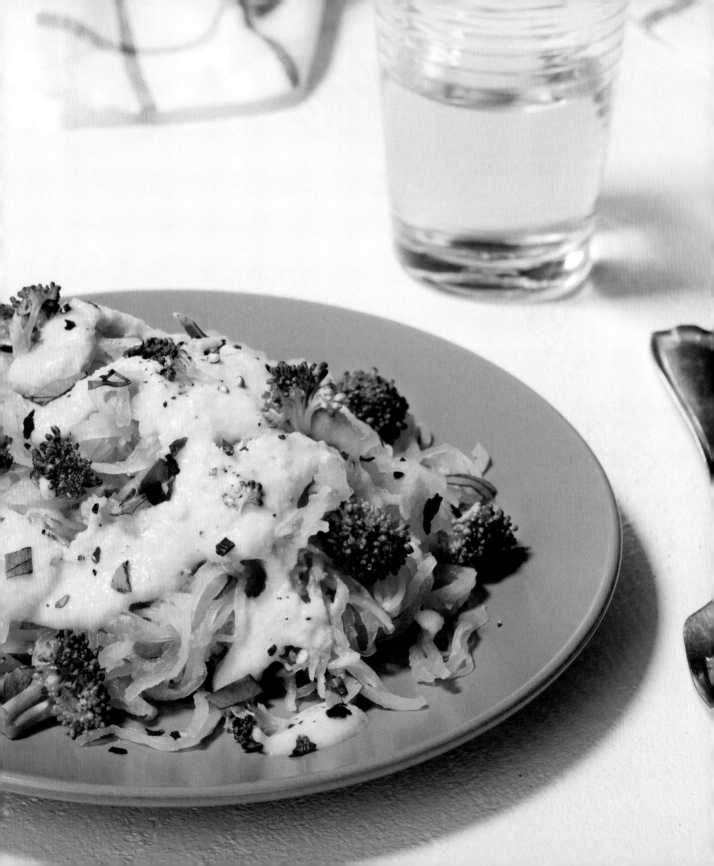

spaghetti squash pasta & broccoli with dairy-free alfredo

Prep Time: **20 minutes** | Cook Time: **30 minutes** | Total Time: **50 minutes** | Makes **4 servings**

GF

GrF

DF

EF

V

NAS

1 cup raw cashews (whole or pieces)

2 cups hot water

1 (2½-pound) spaghetti squash

1 tablespoon avocado oil or extra-virgin olive oil

¾ cup unsweetened plain almond milk or unsweetened nondairy milk of choice

2 tablespoons nutritional yeast

1 tablespoon fresh lemon juice (½ lemon)

2 garlic cloves, chopped

1 teaspoon fine salt, plus more as needed

⅛ teaspoon ground black pepper

1½ pounds broccoli florets (5 cups)

¼ cup loosely packed fresh basil leaves, roughly chopped

Crushed red pepper flakes (optional)

Tips from the Dietitians

A high-powered blender will give you the best results when making the Alfredo sauce.

This recipe also tastes great topped with cooked shrimp or chicken, which adds a boost of protein. To keep it vegan, you could use cubes of cooked tofu instead.

This dish is based on one of the most popular recipes on our website. We swap the traditional cream sauce for one made from cashews, and the pasta for silky strands of spaghetti squash to make a lightened-up version of a comfort food classic.

Preheat the oven to 400°F.

In a small bowl, combine the cashews and hot water. Set aside to soak for 30 minutes while you prepare the remaining ingredients, then drain.

Meanwhile, cut the squash in half lengthwise with a large knife. Using a spoon, scoop out and discard the seeds. Brush the cut sides of the squash with the avocado oil and place it cut side down on a baking sheet. Roast for 30 to 35 minutes, or until the squash is tender and easily pierced with a fork.

While the squash is roasting, make the sauce: In a blender (see Tips), combine the cashews with the nondairy milk, nutritional yeast, lemon juice, garlic, salt, and black pepper. Blend until smooth. Taste, and add more salt, if needed.

Bring a cup of water to a boil in a medium saucepan with a steamer basket set inside. Add the broccoli to the steamer basket, cover, and steam for 4 to 6 minutes, or until the broccoli is cooked to your desired texture.

Remove the squash from the oven, and once cooled enough to handle, use a fork to scrape out the strands and transfer them to a large skillet over medium heat; discard the rinds.

Add the Alfredo sauce and broccoli to the skillet and cook, tossing gently with tongs, until the sauce is heated through, 3 to 5 minutes. Top with the basil and crushed red pepper flakes, if using, and serve.

Store leftovers in an airtight container in the refrigerator for up to 4 days.

Nutrition Info: (Serving size: about 1⅓ cups) 301 calories, 17g total fat, 3g saturated fat, 703mg sodium, 20g carbs, 12g sugar, 5g fiber, 12g protein

sweet potato & black bean burrito bowls

Prep Time: **20 minutes** | Cook Time: **30 minutes** | Total Time: **50 minutes** | Makes **4 servings**

FOR THE BOWLS

1 cup uncooked long-grain white rice (such as basmati; see Tips)

2 cups water

¾ teaspoon fine salt, divided

1 medium to large sweet potato (10 to 12 ounces), peeled and cut into ½-inch cubes (2 to 2½ cups)

½ medium red onion, chopped (1 cup)

2 tablespoons avocado oil or extra-virgin olive oil

1 teaspoon chili powder

½ teaspoon dried oregano

2 cups bite-size cauliflower florets (5 ounces or ½ small head)

1 (4-ounce) can diced or chopped green chiles with their liquid

1 (15-ounce) can black beans, drained and rinsed

½ cup loosely packed fresh cilantro leaves, roughly chopped

1 lime, cut into 4 wedges, for serving

FOR THE CREMA

½ cup sour cream or plain Greek yogurt (use a nondairy version for dairy-free and vegan)

2 tablespoons fresh lime juice (1 medium lime)

¼ teaspoon garlic powder

¼ teaspoon ground cumin

¼ teaspoon fine salt

While this burrito bowl is a meal in itself, don't let that stop you from getting creative and taking it over the top (in a good way). We like to serve these bowls with a side of our vibrant, crunchy Cilantro-Lime Slaw (page 58), and topped with our Loaded Guacamole (page 203), homemade Six-Ingredient Pico De Gallo (page 263), and life-changing Quick-Pickled Onions (page 265) to create a Mexican-inspired feast at home, where guac is never extra! Want to keep it simple? Serve the bowls with sliced avocado, fresh cilantro, and your favorite salsa.

For the bowls: Preheat the oven to 400°F. Line a rimmed baking sheet with parchment paper.

Place the rice in a fine-mesh strainer and rinse under cold running water, then drain. Transfer to a small saucepan, then add the water and ¼ teaspoon of the salt. Bring to a boil, then decrease the heat to low, cover, and simmer without lifting the lid until the rice is tender and almost all of the water is absorbed, 15 to 17 minutes. Remove the saucepan from the heat and let stand, covered, for 10 minutes. Fluff with a fork and set aside.

Meanwhile, place the sweet potato and onion on the prepared baking sheet. In a small bowl, combine the avocado oil, chili powder, oregano, and the remaining ½ teaspoon salt. Whisk to combine. Drizzle half of the oil mixture over the sweet potato and onion and toss to coat.

Bake for 12 minutes, then remove the baking sheet from the oven.

Add the cauliflower and diced chiles with their liquid to the baking sheet along with the remaining oil mixture. Stir gently, then spread into a single layer and bake for 10 minutes.

Remove the baking sheet from the oven and add the black beans. Stir gently and bake for 5 to 7 minutes, or until the beans are heated through and the sweet potato and cauliflower are tender.

Optional toppings:
Sliced avocado or Loaded
    Guacamole (page 203),
    Six-Ingredient Pico de Gallo
    (page 263), Cilantro-Lime Slaw
    (page 58), and/or Quick-Pickled
    Onions (page 265)

Meanwhile, make the crema: In a small bowl, combine the sour cream with the lime juice, garlic powder, cumin, and salt and stir well.

Scoop the rice into bowls, then top with the vegetable mixture, cilantro, and crema. Serve with the lime wedges and desired toppings.

Store leftovers in separate airtight containers in the refrigerator for up to 4 days.

Tips from the Dietitians

Missing the meat? We've got you covered with our Instant Pot Beef Barbacoa Burrito Bowls (page 123) or Slow Cooker Tacos al Pastor (page 129). Both are great options to add to your bowl.

Replace the rice with cauliflower rice for a grain-free option.

Nutrition Info: (Serving size: 1 cup vegetables plus 1 cup rice plus 2½ tablespoons crema, without the optional toppings) 454 calories, 14g total fat, 4g saturated fat, 762mg sodium, 70g carbs, 9g sugar, 8g fiber, 14g protein

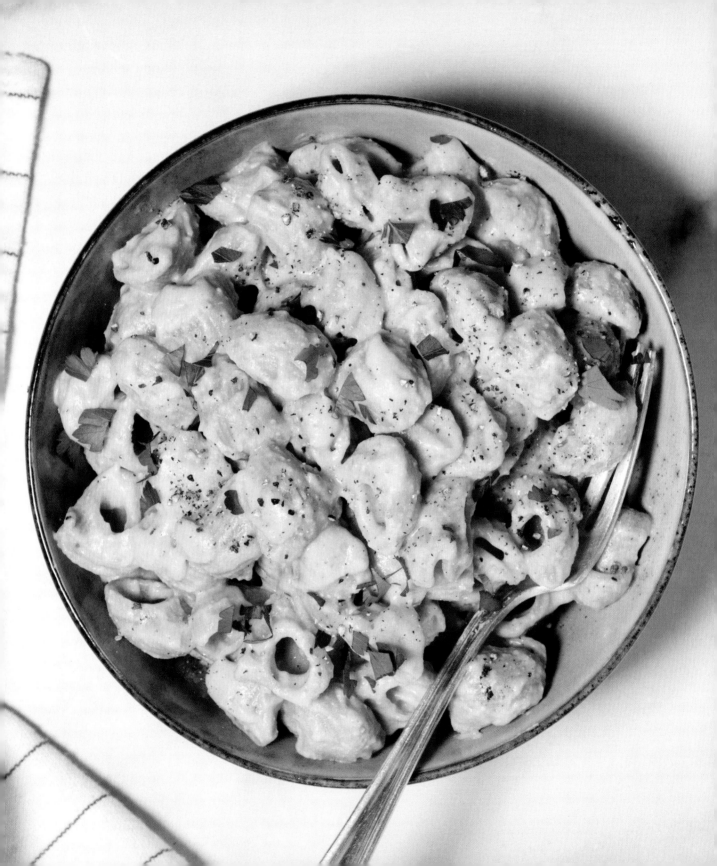

dairy-free mac & "cheese"

Prep Time: **20 minutes** | Cook Time: **15 minutes** | Total Time: **35 minutes** | Makes **6 servings**

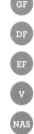

½ cup raw cashews (whole or pieces)

1 cup hot water

1 teaspoon avocado oil or extra-virgin olive oil

½ small yellow onion, diced (½ cup)

3 garlic cloves, minced

¾ teaspoon fine salt, plus more as needed

Ground black pepper

1 small carrot, peeled and diced (½ cup)

2 Yukon Gold potatoes, scrubbed clean and diced (1 cup)

⅔ cup low-sodium vegetable broth or water, plus more as needed

16 ounces gluten-free pasta of choice

⅓ cup unsweetened plain almond milk or unsweetened nondairy milk of choice

2 tablespoons nutritional yeast

1½ tablespoons fresh lemon juice (½ medium lemon)

¾ teaspoon Dijon mustard

Tips from the Dietitians:

This recipe makes 2 cups of "cheese" sauce, which is enough for 16 ounces of pasta. The "cheese" sauce is freezer friendly, so you can use half for 8 ounces of pasta, then freeze the remaining sauce for later.

This ultimate comfort food gets a dairy-free twist! We've hidden veggies in the sauce, but you can keep that secret to yourself if you've got veggie-avoiding family members to feed like we do.

In a small bowl, combine the cashews and hot water. Set aside to soak for 30 minutes while you prepare the remaining ingredients, then drain.

Place a small saucepan over medium-high heat. When hot, add the avocado oil and swirl to coat the bottom. Add the onion and garlic. Season with a dash each of salt and pepper and cook, stirring occasionally, until the onion is softened, 3 to 4 minutes.

To the saucepan, add the carrot, potatoes, and broth. Decrease the heat to low, bring to a gentle simmer, cover, and cook, stirring every 3 to 4 minutes, until the vegetables are tender, 10 to 12 minutes. The vegetables should absorb most of the liquid. Add an additional splash of broth if the liquid has completely dried up.

While the vegetables are cooking, bring a large pot of salted water to a boil. Cook the pasta according to the package directions, then drain.

Drain the vegetables, if necessary, then transfer them to a blender. Add the cashews, almond milk, nutritional yeast, lemon juice, mustard, the ¾ teaspoon salt, and a pinch of pepper. Blend until smooth, scraping down the sides as needed.

Pour the sauce over the pasta and toss to coat evenly. Add salt and pepper to taste. Serve.

Store leftovers in an airtight container in the refrigerator for up to 4 days.

Nutrition Info: (Serving size: 1⅓ cups) 250 calories, 6g total fat, 1g saturated fat, 354mg sodium, 42g carbs, 3g sugar, 3g fiber, 6g protein

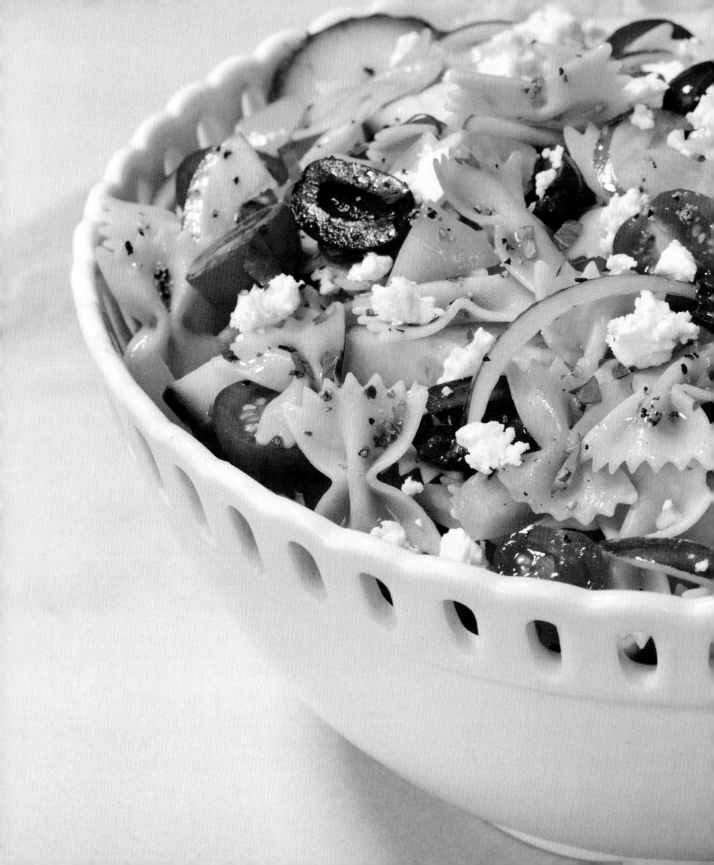

mediterranean pasta salad

Prep Time: **20 minutes** | Cook Time: **15 minutes** | Total Time: **35 minutes** | Makes **12 servings**

GF

DFO

EF

VEG

VO

NAS

Fine salt

8 ounces gluten-free pasta of choice, such as farfalle

1 pint grape tomatoes, halved (2 cups)

1 English cucumber, halved or quartered lengthwise, then sliced ½ inch thick (2 cups)

1 medium bell pepper (any color), diced (1 cup)

½ small red onion, thinly sliced (1 cup)

½ cup pitted kalamata olives, halved

1 cup crumbled feta cheese (omit for dairy-free and vegan)

½ cup loosely packed fresh flat-leaf parsley, roughly chopped

½ cup Greek Vinaigrette and Marinade, plus more as needed (see Tips)

It wouldn't be a cookbook written by a couple of midwesterners if there wasn't a pasta salad in it. This, however, isn't your average church cookbook pasta salad. It's a veggie-loaded, flavor-packed feast for the eyes and taste buds—tasty bits of feta cheese and kalamata olives keep every bite interesting. And the homemade Greek Vinaigrette and Marinade (page 258) is a game changer, if we do say so ourselves. This recipe makes enough to feed a crowd, making it ideal for potlucks, picnics, and backyard barbecues with the neighbors.

Bring a large pot of salted water to a boil. Cook the pasta according to the package directions, then drain well. Allow the pasta to cool while you prepare the other ingredients.

In a large bowl, combine the cooled pasta with the tomatoes, cucumber, bell pepper, red onion, olives, feta cheese, and parsley. Give the vinaigrette a quick stir or shake and add ½ cup to the salad. Toss gently to combine, adding more vinaigrette if needed. Serve.

Store leftovers in an airtight container in the refrigerator for up to 4 days.

Tips from the Dietitians
After storing the pasta salad in the refrigerator, you may need to add more vinaigrette to recoat the pasta and vegetables.

Nutrition Info: (Serving size: 1 cup) 163 calories, 9g total fat, 2g saturated fat, 224mg sodium, 16g carbs, 2g sugar, 1g fiber, 4g protein

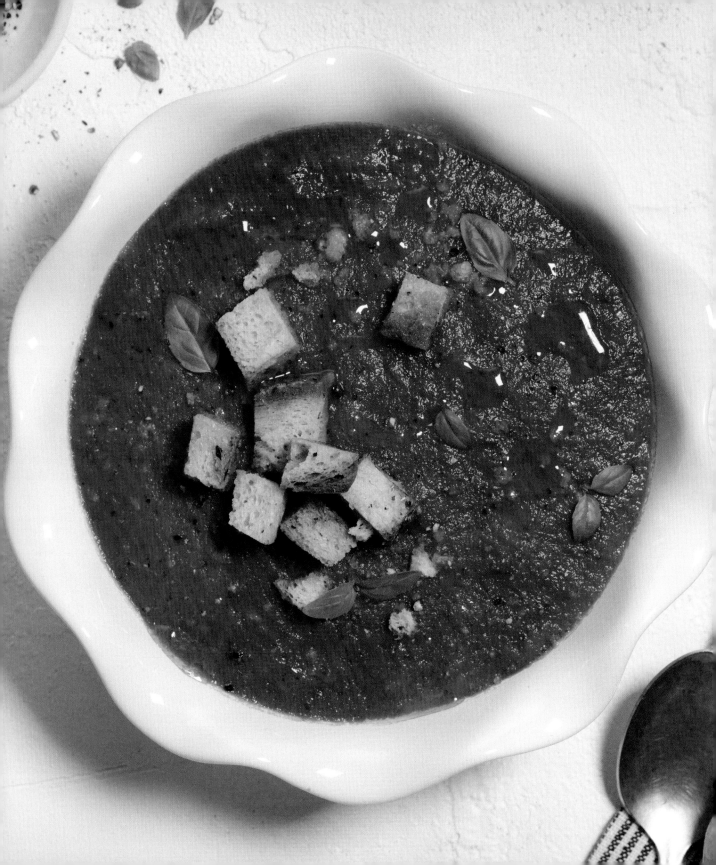

oven-roasted tomato soup

Prep Time: **10 minutes** | Cook Time: **50 minutes** | Total Time: **1 hour** | Makes **4 servings**

GF
DF
EF
V
NF
NAS

FOR THE SOUP
1 (28-ounce) can whole peeled
  tomatoes, drained and juice
  reserved
½ medium yellow onion, thinly
  sliced (1 cup)
3 garlic cloves, slightly smashed
3 tablespoons tomato paste
1½ teaspoons dried basil
½ teaspoon dried thyme
2 tablespoons avocado oil or
  extra-virgin olive oil
2 cups low-sodium vegetable
  broth
Fine salt and ground black pepper

Optional toppings:
Garlic-Herb Croutons, chopped
  fresh basil leaves, and/or grated
  or shaved Parmesan cheese
  (omit for dairy-free and vegan)

Give your next grilled cheese sandwich the love it deserves with a side of homemade tomato soup. Oven roasting canned whole tomatoes with onion, garlic, and tomato paste intensifies the tomato flavor, which adds depth and richness. The Garlic-Herb Croutons (page 269) are optional, but since they're delicious and a great way to make use of leftover bits of bread, we highly recommend them!

Preheat the oven to 375°F. Line a rimmed baking sheet with parchment paper.

Halve the tomatoes if large, then place them on the prepared baking sheet. Add the onion, garlic, tomato paste, basil, and thyme. Drizzle with the avocado oil then stir to combine. Bake for 30 minutes, stirring halfway through.

Remove the baking sheet from the oven. Transfer the roasted tomato mixture to a medium saucepan.

Add the broth and reserved tomato juice to the saucepan. Bring just to a boil then decrease the heat and simmer, uncovered, for 20 minutes.

Blend the soup using an immersion blender or by transferring it to a blender and blending until smooth. Add salt and pepper to taste.

Ladle into bowls and serve with your desired toppings.

Store leftover soup in an airtight container in the refrigerator for up to 4 days or in the freezer for up to 3 months.

> ### Tips from the Dietitians
> This soup freezes well, so consider doubling the recipe using two baking sheets to roast the vegetables and freezing the extra soup for later.

Nutrition Info: (Serving size: 1 cup without the optional toppings) 102 calories, 7g fat, 405mg sodium, 8g carbs, 5g sugar, 6g fiber, 3g protein

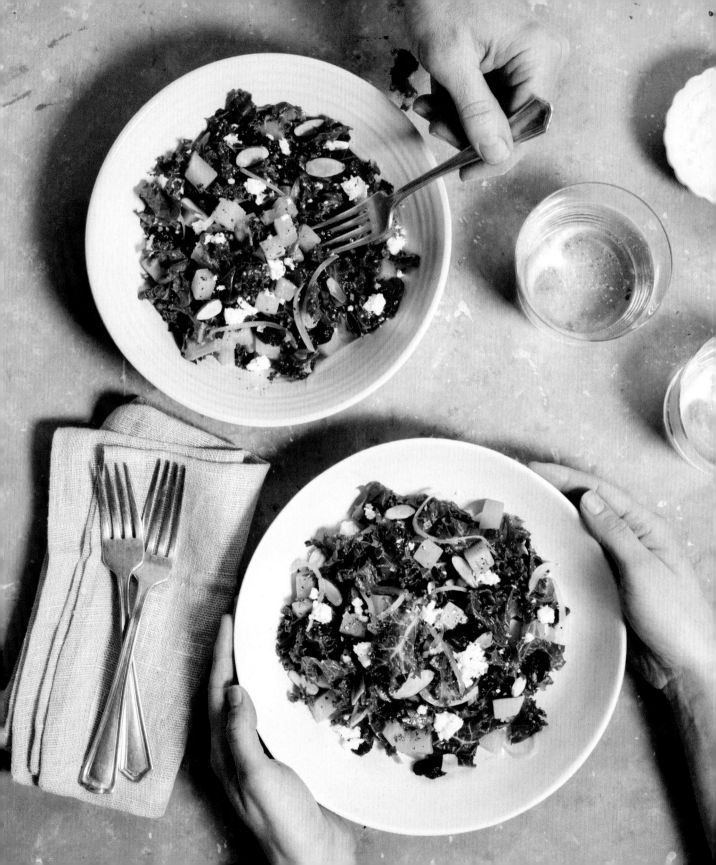

warm butternut squash & kale salad

Prep Time: **20 minutes** | Cook Time: **20 minutes** | Total Time: **40 minutes** | Makes **4 servings**

GF · GrF · DFO · EFO · VEG · VO · NFO · NAS

FOR THE SQUASH AND KALE
- 1 tablespoon avocado oil or extra-virgin olive oil
- 1 (2-pound) butternut squash, peeled and cut into ¼-inch cubes (4 cups; see Tips)
- ¼ cup water
- ¼ cup sliced almonds (or sunflower or pumpkin seeds, for nut-free)
- ¼ cup thinly sliced shallot
- 1 bunch kale, ribs removed and leaves chopped (4 to 5 cups)
- ¼ cup dried cranberries
- ¼ cup soft goat cheese (omit for dairy-free and vegan)

FOR THE DRESSING
- 2 tablespoons fresh lemon juice (½ medium lemon)
- 1 tablespoon avocado oil or extra-virgin olive oil
- ½ teaspoon Dijon mustard
- ¼ teaspoon dried thyme
- Fine salt and ground black pepper

Optional for serving:
- 4 to 8 fried eggs (omit for vegan and egg-free)

Tips from the Dietitians
To save time, buy cubed, peeled butternut squash from the produce section of the grocery store. Cut the cubes into smaller pieces if they're bigger than ¼ inch.

Somewhere between a hash and a warm salad, this combination of sweet winter squash, earthy kale, tart dried cranberries, and creamy goat cheese is a riot of flavors and textures. The light lemony dressing adds just the right amount of tanginess, which will keep you coming back for "just one more bite." Stacie loves to serve this dish with a fried egg (or two!) for a hearty breakfast or meatless lunch.

Start the squash and kale: Place a large skillet over medium-high heat. When hot, add the avocado oil and swirl to coat the bottom. Add the squash and stir to coat with the avocado oil. Add the water to the skillet and cover with a lid. Decrease the heat to medium and cook, stirring occasionally, for 10 minutes.

Place a small skillet over medium heat. When hot, add the almonds and cook, stirring often, until they are golden and give off a toasted aroma, 6 to 8 minutes. Transfer the almonds to a plate to cool.

Meanwhile, make the dressing: In a small bowl, combine the lemon juice, avocado oil, mustard, and thyme and whisk well. Add salt and pepper to taste.

Finish the squash and kale: Add the shallot to the squash in the skillet. Cook, stirring often, until the shallot just starts to soften and the squash is almost tender, 3 to 4 minutes. Add the kale and stir. Cover and cook until the kale is wilted and the squash is tender, 2 to 3 minutes.

Remove the skillet from the heat. Add the almonds and cranberries. Pour the dressing over the salad and toss gently to combine. Transfer the salad to a serving bowl or platter and sprinkle with the goat cheese.

Serve each bowl topped with 1 or 2 fried eggs, if desired.

Store leftovers in an airtight container in the refrigerator for up to 3 days.

Nutrition Info: (Serving size: 1½ cups without the eggs) 229 calories, 11g total fat, 3g saturated fat, 129mg sodium, 32g carbs, 12g sugar, 8g fiber, 5g protein

appetizers,
snacks
& drinks

Ranch Party Mix

Chili-Lime Cowgirl Caviar

Loaded Guacamole

Layered Greek Hummus Dip

Dairy-Free Nacho Cheese

Sticky Teriyaki Chicken Wings

Bacon Ranch Deviled Eggs

Rainbow Veggie Summer Rolls
with Peanut Dipping Sauce

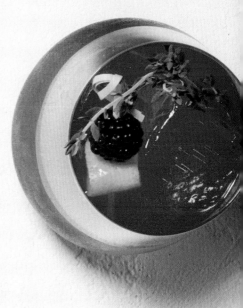

Real Food Margaritas

Summery Strawberry White Sangria

Blackberry-Thyme Vodka Lemonade

Pomegranate Moscow Mules

Mango Daiquiris

Cherry-Lime Mojitos

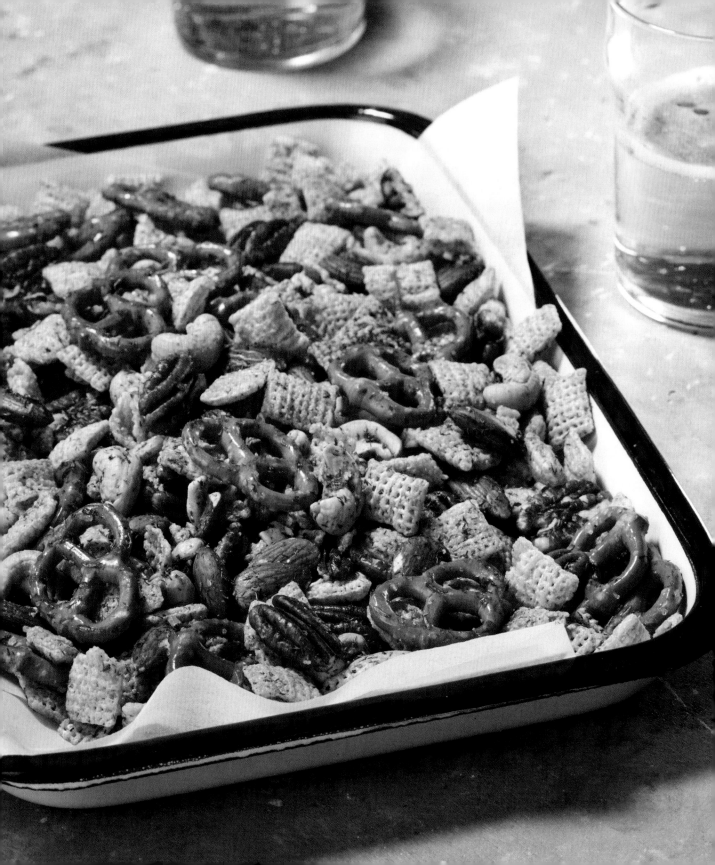

ranch party mix

Prep Time: **10 minutes** | Cook Time: **45 minutes** | Total Time: **55 minutes, plus 20 minutes for cooling** | Makes **14 servings**

GF
DF
EF
V
NAS

6 cups gluten-free square rice cereal, such as Rice Chex

3 cups unsalted or lightly salted mixed nuts of choice (raw or roasted; see Tips)

2 cups gluten-free pretzel twists

⅓ cup avocado oil or extra-virgin olive oil

2½ tablespoons Ranch Seasoning Mix (page 257)

½ teaspoon fine salt

We love a good party mix! But it's not the playlist we're talking about, it's the big bowl of crunchy, salty, savory, and perfectly seasoned mix of pretzels, nuts, and cereal that we're digging. Don't worry, you don't need a party to enjoy this snack mix. It's delicious any time of year and for everyday occasions, like after school, a weekend movie night with the family, or even gifting to friends.

Preheat the oven to 250°F.

In a large bowl, combine the cereal, nuts, and pretzels. Set aside.

In a small bowl, combine the avocado oil, Ranch Seasoning Mix, and salt. Whisk well and pour over the cereal mixture. Toss gently with a rubber spatula until all of the cereal mixture is coated.

Transfer the cereal mixture to a rimmed baking sheet. Bake for about 45 minutes, tossing every 15 minutes, or until the nuts are lightly toasted. Remove from the oven and let the party mix cool completely.

Store leftovers in an airtight container at room temperature for up to 2 weeks.

Tips from the Dietitians
We like to use 1 cup of cashews, 1 cup of almonds, and 1 cup of pecans, but feel free to use your favorite combination of nuts or a can of mixed nuts, if you prefer.

Nutrition Info: (Serving size: ¾ cup) 261 calories, 19g total fat, 3g saturated fat, 320mg sodium, 20g carbs, 2g sugar, 4g fiber, 6g protein

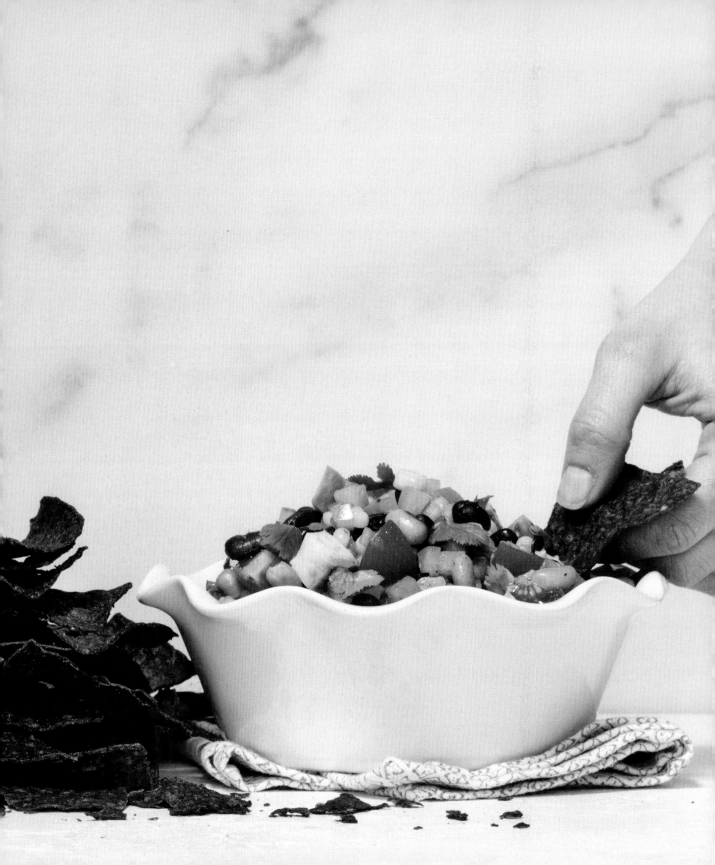

chili-lime cowgirl caviar

Prep Time: **20 minutes** | Total Time: **20 minutes** | Makes **14 servings**

1 (15-ounce) can black-eyed peas, drained and rinsed

1 (15-ounce) can black beans, drained and rinsed

1 (15-ounce) can whole kernel corn, drained and rinsed

1 medium bell pepper (any color), finely diced (1 cup)

1 cup grape tomatoes, diced

½ medium red onion, finely diced (¾ cup)

2 avocados, diced (1½ cups; see Tips)

1 jalapeño, seeds and membranes removed, finely diced (¼ cup; see Tips)

¼ cup loosely packed fresh cilantro leaves, roughly chopped

¼ cup fresh lime juice (2 small limes)

2 tablespoons avocado oil or extra-virgin olive oil

2 tablespoons apple cider vinegar or red wine vinegar

2 teaspoons honey (or agave nectar, for vegan)

1 teaspoon chili powder

½ teaspoon ground cumin

½ teaspoon garlic powder

½ teaspoon salt, plus more as needed

¼ teaspoon ground black pepper

For serving:
Blue corn chips or tortilla chips

While cowboy caviar originated in Texas, we both enjoyed a locally made store-bought version growing up in our home state of Minnesota. This cross between a bean salad and salsa frequently made appearances at holiday family gatherings and weekends at the lake cabin "up north." This is our version that features less oil, a tangy lime dressing spiked with chili powder, a little extra kick from fresh jalapeños, a dose of healthy fat from avocados, and just enough honey to balance the flavors.

In a large bowl, combine the black-eyed peas, black beans, corn, bell pepper, tomatoes, onion, avocado, jalapeño, and cilantro. Set aside.

In a small bowl, combine the lime juice, avocado oil, vinegar, honey, chili powder, ground cumin, garlic powder, salt, and black pepper. Whisk well. Pour the dressing over the ingredients in the large bowl. Toss gently to combine. Taste, and add more salt, if needed.

Serve immediately with chips. Store leftovers in an airtight container in the refrigerator for up to 4 days.

Tips from the Dietitians

If making the dish ahead, wait to dice the avocado, then add it along with the dressing just before serving and toss.

For more heat, include the jalapeño membranes and seeds.

Nutrition Info: (Serving size: ¾ cup without chips) 112 calories, 3g total fat, 0g saturated fat, 105mg sodium, 18g carbs, 3g sugar, 5g fiber, 4g protein

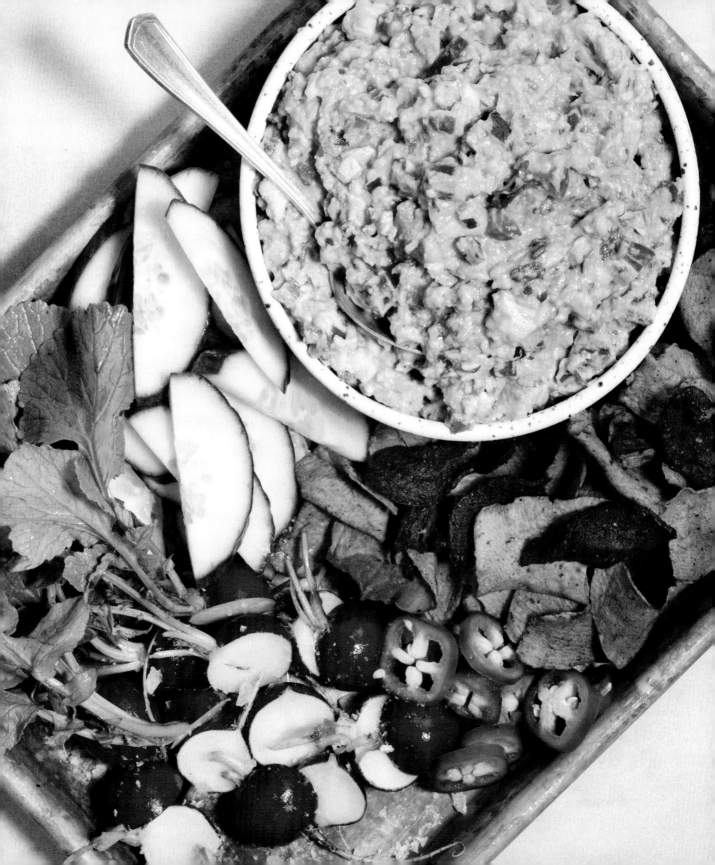

loaded guacamole

Prep Time: **15 minutes** | Total Time: **15 minutes** | Makes **8 servings**

GF
GrF
DF
EF
V
NF
NAS

2 large avocados, peeled or scooped from the skin

⅓ cup finely diced red onion

⅓ cup finely diced bell pepper (any color)

¼ cup loosely packed fresh cilantro leaves, roughly chopped

2 tablespoons fresh lime juice (1 small lime)

2 garlic cloves, minced

½ teaspoon ground cumin

¼ teaspoon fine salt

Optional mix-ins:
Finely diced jalapeño, drained canned black beans, and/or diced tomatoes

For serving:
Blue corn chips or tortilla chips (use a grain-free version or omit for grain-free), plantain chips, sliced cucumbers, sliced jalapeños, halved radishes, and/or vegetable sticks

This is Stacie's recipe for guacamole that she'd been making well before she was a blogger and recipe creator. Family and friends often task her with bringing the guac because it's just so good. It's great served as an appetizer with veggie sticks and, of course, tortilla chips. It's also a tasty accompaniment to any Mexican-inspired meal. Serve it on top of our Sweet Potato and Black Bean Burrito Bowls (page 186), Instant Pot Beef Barbacoa Burrito Bowls (page 123), or Turkey Taco Casserole (page 109).

In a medium bowl, mash the avocados with a fork to your desired consistency. Add the remaining ingredients and mix until combined.

Serve the guacamole with chips and/or vegetable sticks.

Store leftovers in an airtight container in the refrigerator for up to 2 days. To help prevent the guacamole from browning, see Tips.

Tips from the Dietitians
To minimize browning when storing the guacamole, press a piece of parchment paper or plastic wrap onto the surface, then cover the container with a lid.

Nutrition Info: (Serving size: ¼ cup without the optional mix-ins and accompaniments) 64 calories, 5g total fat, 1g saturated fat, 78mg sodium, 5g carbs, 1g sugar, 3g fiber, 1g protein

layered greek hummus dip

Prep Time: **20 minutes** | Total Time: **20 minutes** | Makes **8 servings**

¾ cup plain hummus (a 10-ounce container if using store-bought)

½ cup plain Greek yogurt

1 tablespoon fresh lemon juice

1 tablespoon extra-virgin olive oil, plus more for drizzling

1 garlic clove, pressed or minced

2 teaspoons chopped fresh dill, plus dill fronds for garnish (optional)

¼ teaspoon dried oregano

Pinch each of fine salt and ground black pepper

¾ cup diced English cucumber

¼ cup sliced or quartered grape tomatoes

¼ cup sliced jarred roasted red peppers

3 tablespoons sliced or diced kalamata olives

¼ cup crumbled feta cheese

2 green onions, trimmed and sliced

Cracked black pepper (optional)

For serving:

Vegetable sticks or slices and/ or gluten-free or grain-free crackers

Layers of Greek-inspired goodness come together fast to make this crowd-pleasing dip. We top store-bought hummus with a garlic-lemon yogurt sauce, tomatoes, cucumber, fresh dill, roasted red peppers, kalamata olives, and salty feta cheese. The result is a flavor-packed appetizer or afternoon snack and the perfect accompaniment for fresh veggie sticks and slices or your favorite crackers. Don't be surprised if you can't stop dipping, but if you do have any leftovers, it's delicious spooned onto a salad or added to a wrap or sandwich in place of the usual dressing, mayo, or mustard.

In a 9×9-inch baking dish or similar size platter or plate, spread the hummus evenly onto the bottom.

In a medium bowl, mix the yogurt, lemon juice, olive oil, garlic, dill, oregano, salt, and ground black pepper. Layer the yogurt sauce evenly over the hummus.

Top the yogurt sauce evenly with the cucumber, followed by the tomatoes, red peppers, olives, feta, and green onions. Drizzle lightly with extra-virgin olive oil and top with cracked black pepper and fresh dill, if desired.

Serve with veggies and/or crackers.

Store leftovers in an airtight container in the refrigerator for up to 3 days.

Tips from the Dietitians

To make ahead, we recommend prechopping the ingredients and making the yogurt sauce, then store them separately in airtight containers in the refrigerator for up to 2 days. Just before serving, assemble the layers.

Nutrition Info: (Serving size: about ⅓ cup dip) 97 calories, 6g total fat, 1g saturated fat, 254mg sodium, 7g carbs, 3g sugar, 1g fiber, 3g protein

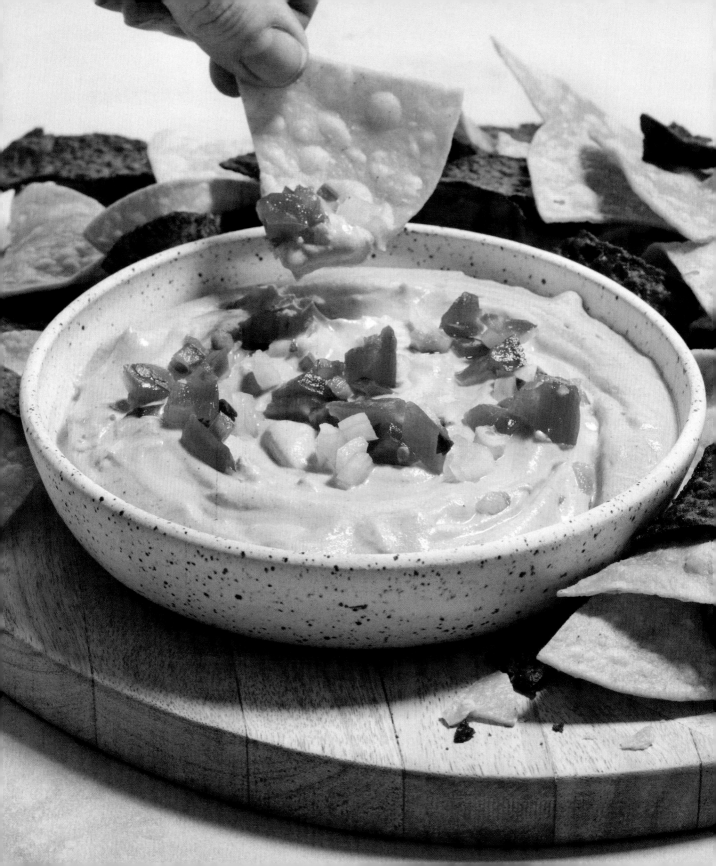

dairy-free nacho cheese

Prep Time: **20 minutes** | Cook Time: **15 minutes** | Total Time: **35 minutes** | Makes **8 servings**

GF
GrF
DF
EF
V
NAS

½ cup raw cashews (whole or
  pieces)
1 cup hot water
1 teaspoon avocado oil or extra-
  virgin olive oil
½ small yellow onion, diced
3 garlic cloves, minced
Fine salt and ground black pepper
1 medium carrot, peeled and diced
1 medium Yukon Gold potato,
  scrubbed clean and diced
⅔ cup low-sodium vegetable broth
  or water, plus more as needed
2 tablespoons unsweetened plain
  almond milk or unsweetened
  nondairy milk of choice
2 tablespoons nutritional yeast
1 tablespoon fresh lime juice
  (1 small lime)
¾ teaspoon chili powder
½ teaspoon smoked paprika
1 (4-ounce) can diced mild green
  chiles, drained

For serving:
Tortilla chips (use a grain-free
  version or omit for grain-free)
  and/or vegetable sticks

Tips from the Dietitians

Want to spice things up? Add a pinch of ancho chile powder or cayenne pepper.

Stir a little of our Six-Ingredient Pico de Gallo (page 263) into the nacho cheese for a restaurant-style queso dip.

This is a dairy-free and vegan version of the delicious queso we get at our favorite Mexican restaurants. The recipe starts with a base of vegetables (yes, vegetables!) and cashews, which blend into the creamiest sauce. We love to drizzle this nacho "cheese" over burrito bowls or serve it as a stand-alone dip with tortilla chips and fresh veggies for dunking.

In a small bowl, combine the cashews and hot water. Set aside to soak for 30 minutes while you prepare the remaining ingredients, then drain.

Place a small saucepan over medium-high heat. When hot, add the avocado oil and swirl to coat the bottom. Add the onion and garlic. Season with a dash of salt and pepper and cook, stirring occasionally, until the onion is softened, 3 to 4 minutes.

To the saucepan, add the carrot, potato, and broth. Turn the heat down to low, bring to a gentle simmer, cover, and cook, stirring every 3 to 4 minutes, until the vegetables are tender, 10 to 12 minutes. The vegetables should absorb most of the liquid. Add an additional splash of broth if the liquid has completely dried up before the vegetables are tender.

Drain the vegetables, if necessary, then transfer them to a blender. Add the cashews, almond milk, nutritional yeast, lime juice, chili powder, paprika, and ½ teaspoon salt. Blend until smooth, scraping down the sides as needed. Taste and add more salt, if needed. Stir in the chiles.

Serve warm, with tortilla chips and vegetable sticks.

Store leftovers in an airtight container in the refrigerator for up to 4 days.

Nutrition Info: (Serving size: ¼ cup without chips and vegetable sticks) 103 calories, 4g total fat, 1g saturated fat, 127mg sodium, 16g carbs, 4g sugar, 2g fiber, 3g protein

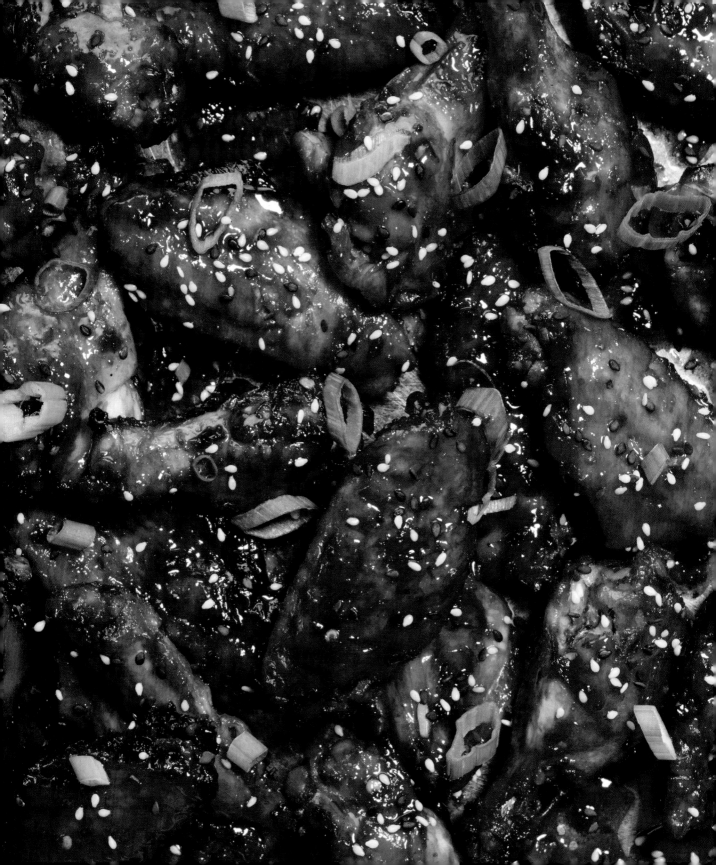

sticky teriyaki chicken wings

Prep Time: **10 minutes** | Cook Time: **1 hour** | Total Time: **1 hour 10 minutes** | Makes **8 servings as an appetizer (or 4 servings as a meal)**

Nonstick cooking spray

3 pounds chicken wings, flats and drumettes separated, tips discarded (see Tips)

⅓ cup coconut aminos

3 tablespoons honey

1 tablespoon rice vinegar or apple cider vinegar

1 teaspoon toasted sesame oil

2 garlic cloves, grated or finely minced

1 teaspoon grated peeled fresh ginger (1-inch piece)

½ teaspoon crushed red pepper flakes (optional)

Optional toppings:
Green onions, white and green parts, thinly sliced, and/or sesame seeds

Tips from the Dietitians
If your wings are whole, you'll need to separate them into flats and drumettes, and cut off the wing tips before using them in this recipe. Save the wing tips for making broth or cooking in a batch of our Homestyle Chicken and Rice Soup (page 92).

All we can say is, "OMG!" (with our mouths full) because these wings are so ridiculously delicious and hard to stop eating once you start. The homemade teriyaki sauce takes just minutes to make and, at first glance, seems underwhelming, but trust the process. The magic happens in the oven, resulting in sticky-sweet wings that will have you licking your fingers. We use coconut aminos instead of soy sauce to make them soy-free and to reduce the amount of sodium. These wings can also be served as a meal with Coconut-Lime Rice (page 71), Crispy Broccoli (page 70), and a side of Quick-Pickled Carrots or Cucumbers (page 267).

Preheat the oven to 425°F. Spray a 9×13-inch baking dish with cooking spray.

Place the chicken wing flats and drumettes in the prepared baking dish.

In a small bowl, combine the coconut aminos, honey, vinegar, sesame oil, garlic, ginger, and crushed red pepper flakes, if using. Whisk well to combine. Pour over the chicken wings and toss to coat completely. Arrange the wings in a single layer as much as possible.

Bake for 30 minutes. Flip the wings and rotate the baking dish, then bake for about another 30 minutes, or until the sauce is sticky and the wings are browned a bit.

Remove from the oven. Sprinkle the wings with green onions and/or sesame seeds, if desired, and serve.

Store leftovers in an airtight container in the refrigerator for up to 3 days.

Nutrition Info: (Serving size: 4 pieces without the optional toppings) 354 calories, 22g total fat, 6g saturated fat, 321mg sodium, 9g carbs, 8g sugar, 0g fiber, 30g protein

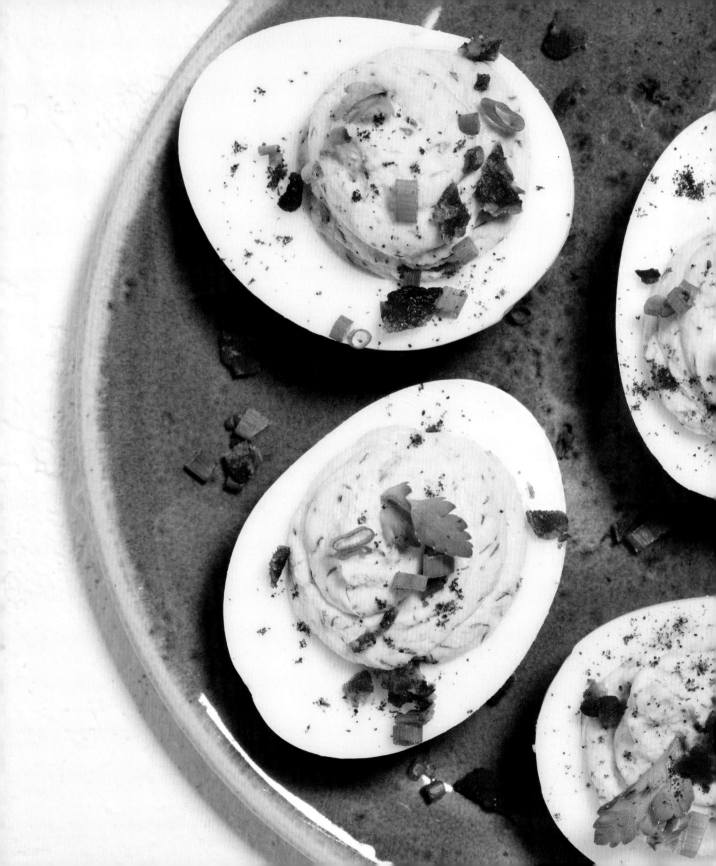

bacon ranch deviled eggs

Prep Time: **30 minutes** | Total Time: **30 minutes** | Makes **12 deviled egg halves (6 servings)**

2 thin bacon slices (see Tips)

6 hard-boiled eggs, cooled and peeled (see Easy-Peel Hard-Boiled Eggs; instructions follow)

¼ cup Dairy-Free Ranch Dressing and Dip (or store-bought ranch dressing; see Tips)

1 tablespoon mayonnaise (see Tips)

1 tablespoon chopped fresh chives or parsley, plus more for garnish

1 teaspoon Dijon mustard

Fine salt and ground black pepper

Sweet or smoked paprika, for garnish

We made the classic deviled egg recipe extra flavorful by adding crispy bits of bacon and our delicious Dairy-Free Ranch Dressing and Dip (page 254). If you don't need the recipe to be dairy free, then go ahead and use store-bought ranch dressing. These deviled eggs make an incredibly tasty appetizer or satisfying high-protein snack. Included in this recipe is our secret to making the eggs easy to peel.

Place a small skillet over medium-high heat. When hot, add the bacon and cook until crisp, 2 to 3 minutes per side. Remove the bacon to a paper towel–lined plate. Let cool, then chop or crumble into small pieces. Set aside.

Meanwhile, cut the eggs in half lengthwise. Using a spoon, carefully remove the yolks and place them in a medium bowl. Place the egg whites on a plate and set aside.

To the yolks, add the ranch dressing, mayonnaise, chives, mustard, and 2 tablespoons of the chopped bacon (reserve the rest for garnish) and stir until well combined and smooth. Add salt and pepper to taste.

Spoon 2 to 3 teaspoons of the yolk mixture into each egg white half. Garnish with the chives, the reserved chopped bacon, and a dusting of paprika.

Store any leftovers in an airtight container in the refrigerator for up to 3 days.

To Make Easy-Peel Hard-Boiled Eggs

Fill a medium pot ¾ full with water and bring to a gentle boil.

Make sure the water isn't at a vigorous boil, which may cause the eggs to crack. Adjust the heat, if necessary, then add 1 egg at a time with a slotted spoon. You can cook up to 9 eggs at a time in a medium pot.

Continued on the next page

Set a timer for 12 minutes.

While the eggs are boiling, prepare an ice bath by filling a medium bowl halfway with ice and water.

Once the boiling time is up, immediately transfer the eggs to the ice bath with the slotted spoon and let them cool for 10 minutes.

Peel the eggs.

Store peeled eggs in an airtight container in the refrigerator for up to 3 days. Unpeeled eggs may be stored in the refrigerator for up to 1 week.

Tips from the Dietitians

If you're looking to avoid added sugars, use bacon, ranch dressing, and mayonnaise made without added sugar.

Nutrition Info: (Serving size: 2 deviled egg halves) 149 calories, 12g total fat, 3g saturated fat, 225mg sodium, 1g carbs, 1g sugar, 0g fiber, 7g protein

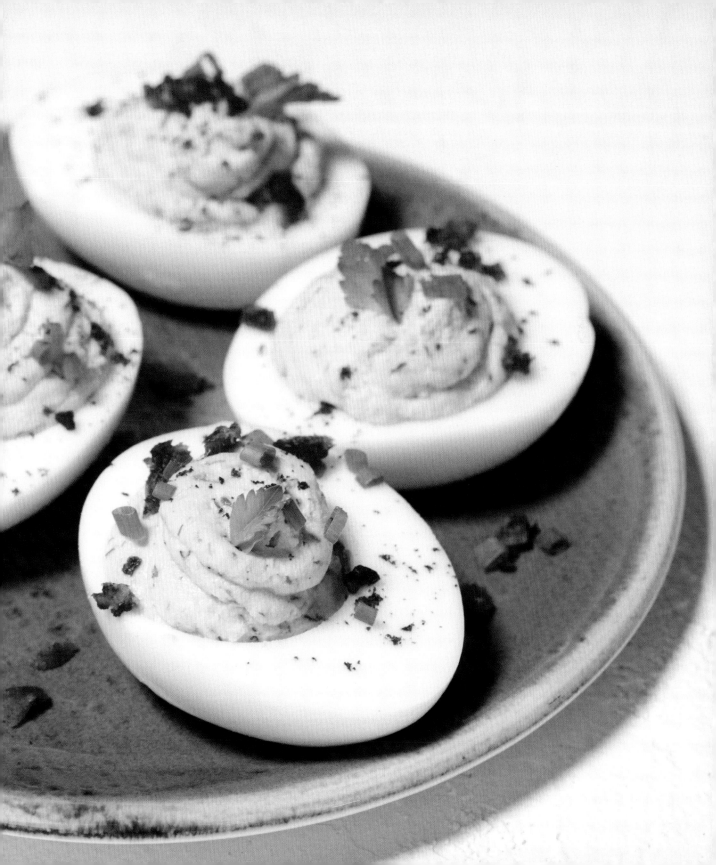

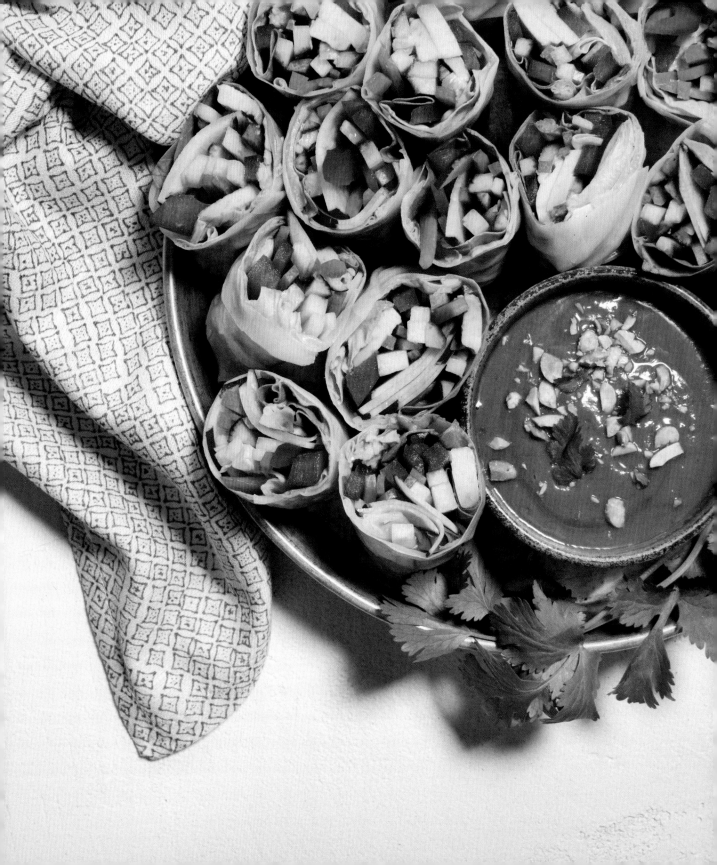

rainbow veggie summer rolls with peanut dipping sauce

Prep Time: **30 minutes** | Total Time: **30 minutes** | Makes **4 servings**

8 (10-inch) rice paper wrappers

8 butter lettuce leaves (or 4 green leaf lettuce leaves, cut in half lengthwise)

1 large avocado, sliced

½ English cucumber, sliced into matchsticks (¾ cup)

1 medium carrot, peeled and sliced into matchsticks (¾ cup)

1 small red bell pepper, thinly sliced (¾ cup)

½ cup sliced radishes or thinly sliced purple cabbage

¼ cup loosely packed fresh cilantro or basil leaves, roughly chopped (or a combination of both)

8 tablespoons Peanut Dressing and Dipping Sauce

On a mission to eat more veggies? Forgo that ho-hum plate of carrots and celery and make these instead. Inspired by Vietnamese spring rolls, which are usually stuffed with vermicelli and shrimp, we've adapted them to have an all-vegetable filling using what's in our crisper, and added creamy avocado to balance the crunch. The Peanut Dressing and Dipping Sauce (page 261) takes this snack over the top.

Assemble one summer roll at a time: Fill a shallow dish (that's large enough to fit the rice paper) with cool water. Working with one sheet at a time, lay the rice paper in the water, pressing down lightly to submerge it fully, 10 to 15 seconds. Transfer the rice paper to a cutting board and lay it flat.

Place 1 butter lettuce leaf (or 2 green leaf lettuce halves) in the center of the rice paper. Top the lettuce with 1 or 2 avocado slices and a few pieces each of cucumber, carrot, bell pepper, radish, and cilantro.

Wrap the summer roll like a burrito: Fold the side of the rice paper nearest to you tightly over the filling. Then fold the left and right sides over the filling and carefully roll the wrapped filling away from you. Cover the roll with a damp paper towel. Continue assembling the rolls with the remaining rice papers and filling.

With a sharp knife, cut each roll in half and serve with the Peanut Dipping Sauce.

Store leftovers in an airtight container in the refrigerator for up to 2 days.

Nutrition Info: (Serving size: 2 rolls with 2 tablespoons dipping sauce) 240 calories, 13g total fat, 2g saturated fat, 316mg sodium, 30g carbs, 7g sugar, 5g fiber, 6g protein

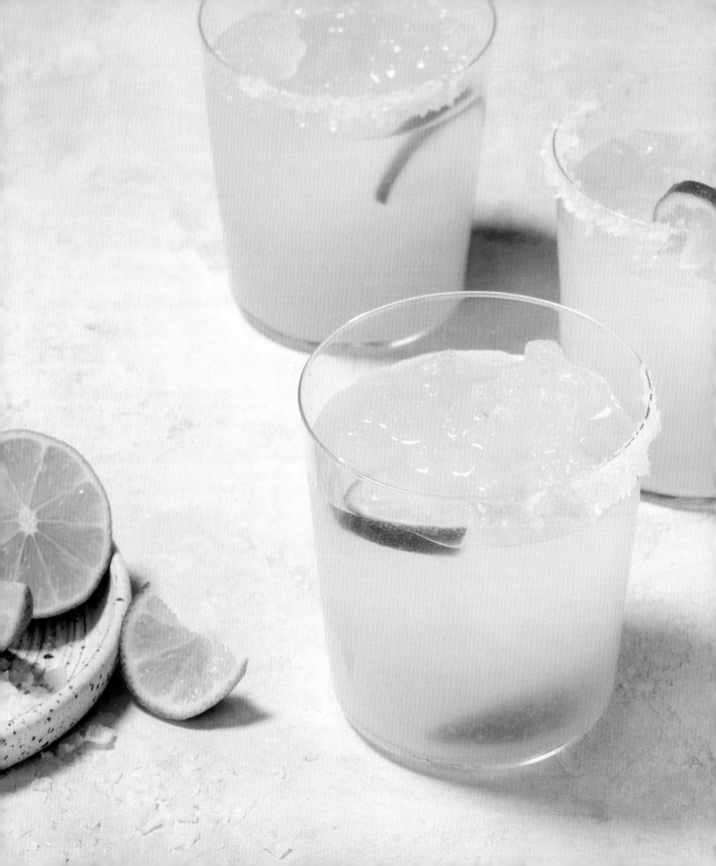

real food margaritas

Prep Time: **15 minutes** | Total Time: **15 minutes** | Makes **4 servings**

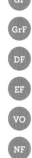

¾ cup fresh lime juice (1 pound limes)

⅓ cup fresh orange juice (1 medium orange)

2 teaspoons honey (or agave nectar, for vegan)

1 cup tequila (blanco or reposado)

2 cups unsweetened coconut water

¼ cup coarse salt, for rimming the glasses (optional)

5 lime wedges or slices, for rimming and for garnish (optional)

Ice

Chilled sparkling water, for topping

We love a good margarita, but what we don't love is the sugar crash that comes from syrupy sweet premade mixers. Our lower-sugar take on this popular drink uses fresh citrus juice, coconut water, and just a touch of natural sweetener to create a refreshing cocktail. The next time life gives you limes, or tacos are on the menu, make a batch of these margaritas!

Combine the lime juice and orange juice in a pitcher or quart-size mason jar. Add the honey and stir until dissolved. Add the tequila and coconut water and stir to combine.

If rimming the glasses with salt: Place the salt in a small, shallow dish. Rub a lime wedge or lime slice around the rim of each of four old-fashioned glasses or pint-size jars, then invert each glass into the salt and gently twist back and forth a few times to coat the rim.

Fill the glasses with ice and divide the margarita mixture evenly among them. Top off each glass with sparkling water, and garnish with a lime slice or wedge, if using, and serve immediately.

Nutrition Info: (Serving size:1 drink without the salted rim) 176 calories, 0g total fat, 0g saturated fat, 31mg sodium, 12g carbs, 9g sugar, 0g fiber, 0g protein

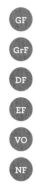

summery strawberry white sangria

Prep Time: **15 minutes** | Total Time: **15 minutes, plus 2 hours for chilling** | Makes **6 servings**

⅔ cup fresh lemon juice
(3 to 4 medium lemons)
⅔ cup fresh orange juice
(2 medium oranges)
3 tablespoons honey (or agave
nectar, for vegan)
1 pound fresh strawberries, hulled
and sliced, divided
1 (750ml) bottle chilled dry white
wine, such as pinot grigio or
sauvignon blanc
2 cups chilled sparkling water
Ice, for serving (optional)
1 lemon, sliced into 6 rounds
6 fresh mint sprigs, for garnish

Sangria is a delicious way to highlight the best of what's in season. Here we combine plump sweet strawberries with fresh citrus juice, dry white wine, and a touch of honey for a grown-up version of strawberry lemonade. Adding a splash of sparkling water makes this white sangria especially light and refreshing, so it's perfect for summertime sipping.

In a blender, combine the lemon juice, orange juice, honey, and half of the strawberries, and blend until smooth. Pour, a little at a time, through a fine-mesh sieve into a pitcher or half-gallon jar. Discard any solids left in the sieve.

Stir the wine and remaining strawberries into the pitcher. Cover and refrigerate until the sangria is cold, up to 24 hours.

Just before serving, gently stir the sparkling water into the pitcher.

Pour the sangria into large wineglasses with a few ice cubes, if desired, and garnish each with a lemon slice and mint sprig. Serve immediately.

Nutrition Info: (Serving size: 1 drink) 162 calories, 0g total fat, 0g saturated fat, 10mg sodium, 17g carbs, 13g sugar, 1g fiber, 1g protein

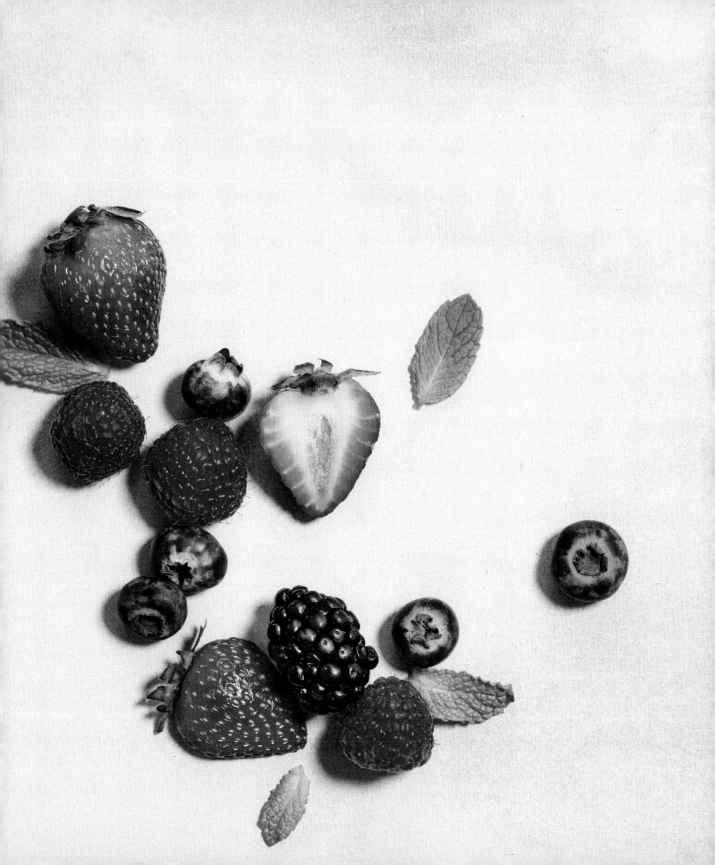

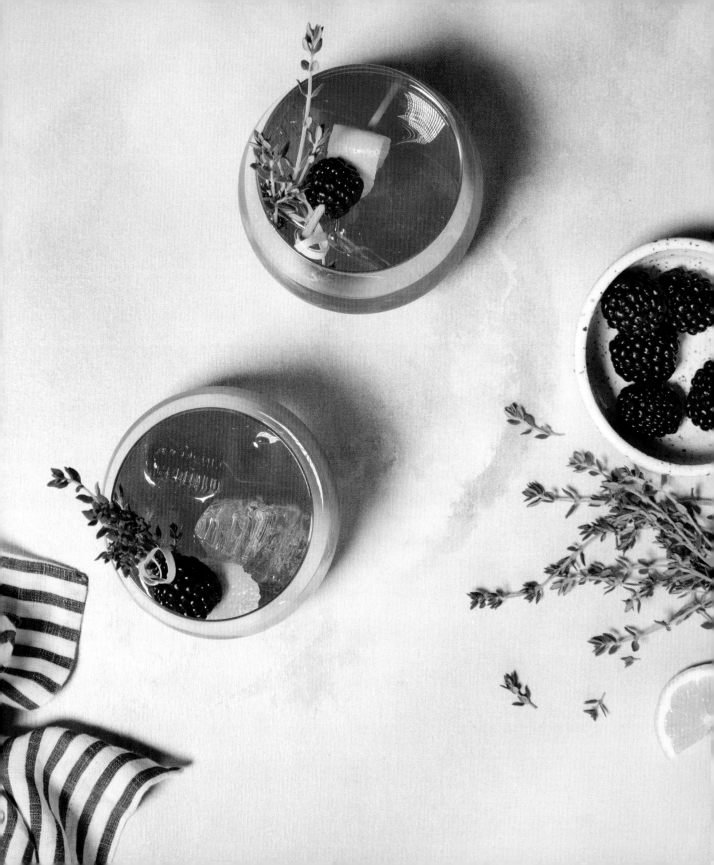

blackberry-thyme vodka lemonade

Prep Time: **10 minutes** | Cook Time: **5 minutes** | Total Time: **15 minutes, plus 1 hour for cooling** | Makes **4 servings**

GF
GrF
DF
EF
VO
NF

¼ cup honey (or agave nectar, for vegan)
¼ cup water
Grated zest of 2 lemons
12 fresh thyme sprigs
1 cup fresh blackberries, divided
¾ cup fresh lemon juice (3 to 4 medium lemons)
Ice
1 cup vodka
Chilled sparkling water, for topping

Optional garnishes:
4 lemon slices and/or 4 fresh thyme sprigs

Tips from the Dietitians
The thyme-infused honey can be made up to 3 days in advance and kept in the refrigerator until ready to use.

For a nonalcoholic version of this cocktail, omit the vodka and add an extra splash of sparkling water when topping the drink.

While this cocktail takes a little more work to make, it's definitely worth the effort. Instead of sweetening the drink with a traditional simple syrup, we infuse honey with herbaceous thyme and sweet-tart blackberries. It creates the base for a one-of-a-kind drink that you'll want to make again and again.

Combine the honey, water, and lemon zest in a small saucepan. Bring just to a boil, then remove from the heat.

Gently crush or bruise the 12 thyme sprigs between your fingers to help release some of the fragrant oil from the leaves. Drop the thyme sprigs into the honey mixture, stir, and allow to cool in the saucepan for 1 hour (see Tips).

Once the thyme-infused honey has cooled, add ¾ cup of the blackberries to the saucepan (reserve the rest for garnish). Using a fork or potato masher, mash the berries to release their juice.

Pour the berry-honey mixture through a fine-mesh sieve into a medium bowl. Discard any solids left in the sieve. Add the lemon juice and stir.

Fill four old-fashioned or double highball glasses about ¾ full with ice. Divide the berry lemonade among the glasses.

To each glass, add ¼ cup of the vodka, top it off with sparkling water, and stir gently to mix; garnish with the reserved blackberries and a lemon slice and/or a sprig of thyme, if desired. Serve immediately.

Nutrition Info: (Serving size: 1 drink) 216 calories, 0g fat, 0g saturated fat, 2mg sodium, 24g carbs, 19g sugar, 2g fiber, 1g protein

pomegranate moscow mules

Prep Time: **10 minutes** | Total Time: **10 minutes** | Makes **4 servings**

GF
GrF
DF
EF
V
NF

Ice
1 cup unsweetened pomegranate
    juice
8 tablespoons fresh lime juice
    (3 medium limes)
8 ounces gluten-free vodka (or
    a splash of chilled sparkling
    water, for nonalcoholic)
16 ounces ginger kombucha (or
    ginger beer)
8 tablespoons pomegranate
    seeds

Optional garnishes:
4 fresh rosemary sprigs and 4 lime
    wedges

Pomegranates are only in season late fall through early winter, which makes them a special treat no matter how you enjoy them. We use them in this Moscow mule twist that's packed with holiday cheer and a healthy dose of antioxidants. Swapping out the usual ginger beer for your favorite ginger kombucha helps lower the sugar content and gives the drink a little probiotic boost. For a nonalcoholic version, simply leave out the vodka and add a splash of sparkling water.

Fill four copper mugs or old-fashioned glasses halfway with ice. To each glass, add ¼ cup of the pomegranate juice, 2 tablespoons of the lime juice, 2 ounces of the vodka, and 4 ounces of the kombucha and stir gently to mix.

Add 2 tablespoons of the pomegranate seeds to each drink. Garnish with a rosemary sprig and a lime wedge, if desired. Serve immediately.

Nutrition Info: (Serving size: ¼ of the recipe) 185 calories, 0g total fat, 0g saturated fat, 16mg sodium, 14g carbs, 12g sugar, 0g fiber, 0g protein

mango daiquiris

Prep Time: **10 minutes** | Total Time: **10 minutes** | Makes **4 servings**

GF
GrF
DF
EF
VO
NF

2 cups frozen mango chunks
¼ cup fresh lime juice (2 small
  limes)
1 teaspoon honey, plus more as
  desired (or agave nectar, for
  vegan)
¾ cup white rum
1 cup ice cubes

Optional garnish:
4 lime slices

If you're looking for the perfect drink to sip on a hot summer day, this mango daiquiri is made with just five simple ingredients and comes together fast. Just toss all of the ingredients into a blender, give it a whirl, and enjoy!

In a blender, combine the mango, lime juice, honey, rum, and ice, and blend on high until smooth. Taste and add more honey, if desired.

Pour the daiquiri into four old-fashioned glasses, and garnish each with a slice of lime, if desired. Serve immediately.

Nutrition Info: (Serving size: ¼ of the recipe) 151 calories, 0g total fat, 0g saturated fat, 13mg sodium, 14g carbs, 8g sugar, 1g fiber, 1g protein

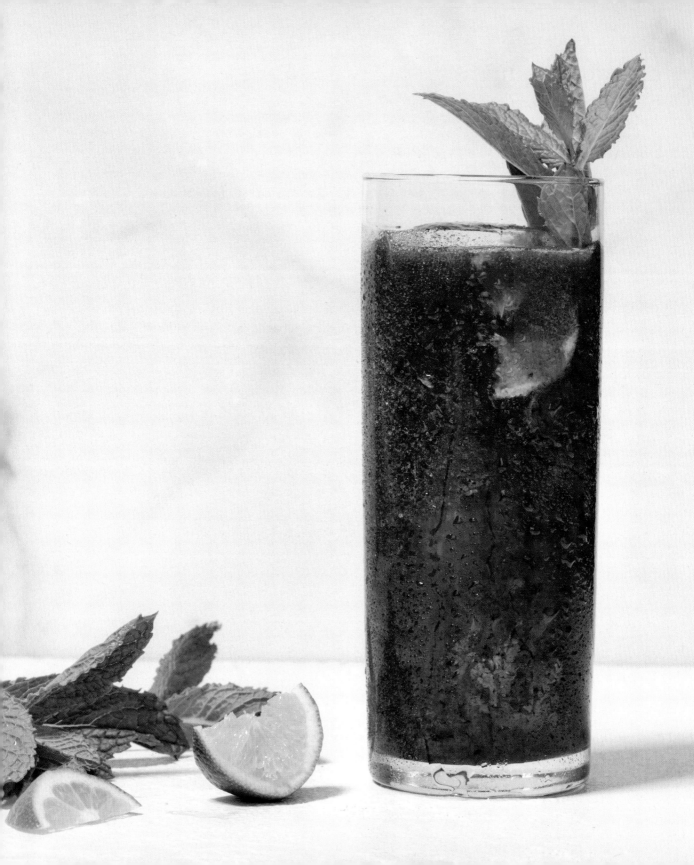

cherry-lime mojitos

Prep Time: **10 minutes** | Total Time: **10 minutes** | Makes **4 servings**

2 cups pitted cherries (thawed, if frozen)

1 tablespoon honey (or agave nectar, for vegan)

30 large or 40 small fresh mint leaves

½ cup fresh lime juice (2-3 medium limes)

Ice

¾ cup white rum

Chilled sparkling water, for topping

Optional garnishes:

4 lime wedges and fresh mint leaves

Cherries and limes come together for a sweet-tart twist on the classic mojito. Fresh cherries are only available for a limited time in the summer, but don't worry, frozen cherries will also work, so you can enjoy this re-fined sugar–free and antioxidant-rich cocktail year-round.

Add the cherries and honey to a blender and blend on high until smooth. Set aside.

Divide the mint leaves and lime juice among four (10- to 14-ounce) tall glasses. With the end of a wooden spoon, muddle (mash) the mint leaves until they begin to release their fragrant oils and the leaves turn dark green.

Fill each glass ¾ of the way with ice. Divide the cherry-honey puree and rum among the four glasses. Stir and top off each glass with sparkling water.

Garnish each glass with a lime wedge and a few fresh mint leaves, if de-sired. Serve immediately.

> **Tips from the Dietitians**
> For a nonalcoholic version of this cocktail, simply leave out the rum and add an extra splash of sparkling water when topping the drink.

GF
GrF
DF
EF
VO
NF

Nutrition Info: (Serving size: 1 drink) 185 calories, 0g total fat, 0g saturated fat, 2mg sodium, 22g carbs, 18g sugar, 2g fiber, 1g protein

desserts & sweet snacks

One-Bowl Mixed Berry Crisp

Jammy Blueberry Pie Bars

Apple Cobbler

Cowgirl Cookies

Peanut Butter Swirl Brownies

One-Bowl Chocolate Chip Blondies

No-Bake Peanut Butter & Jelly Crunch Bites

Trail Mix Granola Bars

No-Bake Energy Bites Three Ways

Easy Fruit Dip Two Ways

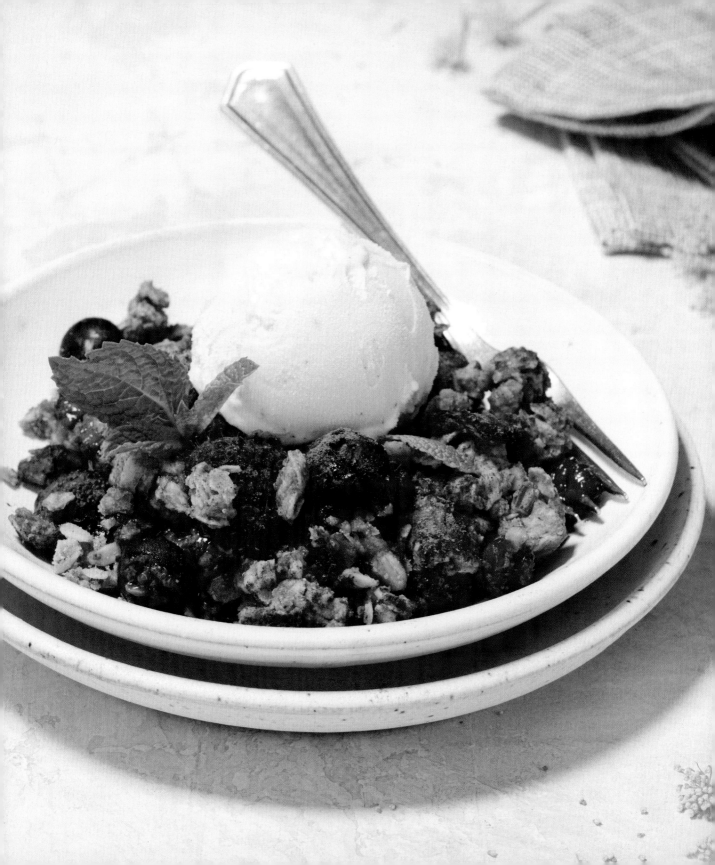

one-bowl mixed berry crisp

Prep Time: **15 minutes** | Cook Time: **35 minutes** | Total Time: **50 minutes, plus 10 minutes for cooling** | Makes **9 servings**

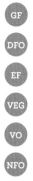

FOR THE FRUIT FILLING
Nonstick cooking spray
5 cups fresh mixed berries (blackberries, blueberries, raspberries, and/or sliced strawberries)
2 tablespoons gluten-free all-purpose flour blend
2 tablespoons pure maple syrup
2 tablespoons water
¼ teaspoon ground cinnamon
Pinch of ground nutmeg

FOR THE CRISP TOPPING
1 cup old-fashioned rolled oats
½ cup gluten-free all-purpose flour blend
¼ cup chopped pecans (omit for nut-free)
¼ cup (4 tablespoons) unsalted butter, melted (use coconut oil or vegan butter, for dairy-free and vegan)
3 tablespoons pure maple syrup
1 teaspoon pure vanilla extract
1 teaspoon ground cinnamon, plus more for dusting
⅛ teaspoon ground nutmeg
Pinch of fine salt

Optional toppings:
Ice cream, whipped cream, vanilla yogurt, nondairy whipped topping (for dairy-free and vegan), and/or fresh mint leaves

When berries are in season you can be sure that we're making the most of those plump, sweet gems by including them in everything from meals to snacks and, of course, desserts. This easy-to-make berry crisp was created with health in mind while making it taste like an indulgent dessert with its fruity filling and perfectly golden crisp topping. Life is too short not to enjoy this ultimate summer dessert with a scoop of your favorite vanilla ice cream!

Preheat the oven to 375°F. Spray a 9x9-inch baking dish with cooking spray.

Make the fruit filling: To the prepared baking dish, add the berries, flour, maple syrup, water, cinnamon, and nutmeg and stir gently to combine. Set aside.

Make the crisp topping: In a medium bowl, combine the oats, flour, pecans, butter, maple syrup, vanilla, cinnamon, nutmeg, and salt and stir well to combine.

Sprinkle the crisp topping evenly over the berry filling, then dust the top with cinnamon. Bake for 30 to 35 minutes, or until bubbly and the top is golden brown.

Remove from the oven and let cool for 10 to 15 minutes.

Serve the crisp warm with your desired topping.

Store leftovers in an airtight container in the refrigerator or at room temperature for up to 3 days.

Nutrition Info: (Serving size: ⅑ of the recipe without the optional toppings) 206 calories, 9g total fat, 4g saturated fat, 23mg sodium, 28g carbs, 13g sugar, 3g fiber, 3g protein

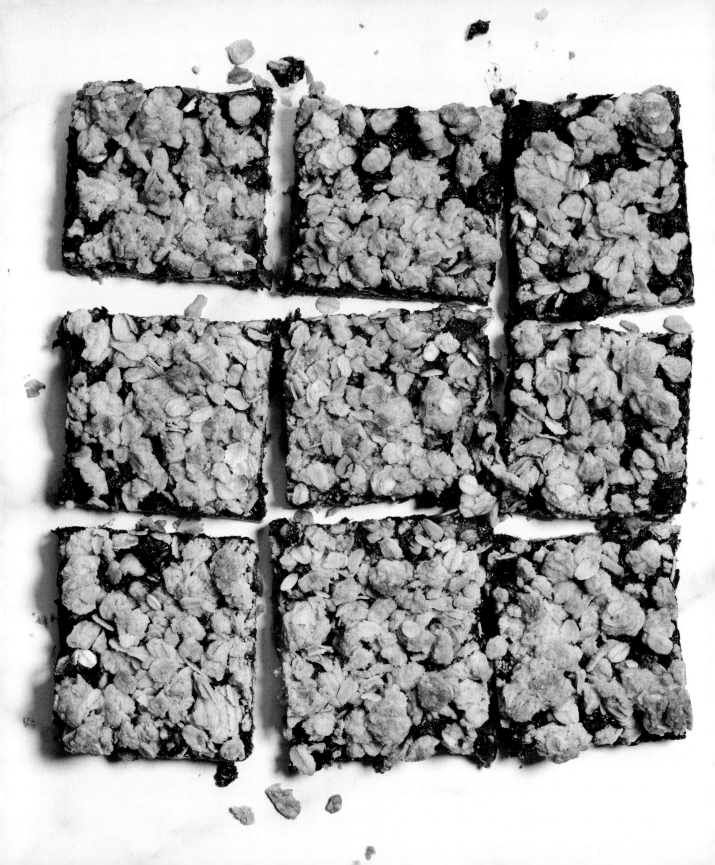

jammy blueberry pie bars

Prep time: **15 minutes** | Cook time: **50 minutes** | Total time: **1 hour 5 minutes, plus 3 hours for cooling and chilling** | Makes **16 bars**

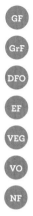

FOR THE CRUST AND TOPPING

1¾ cups old-fashioned rolled oats

¾ cup gluten-free all-purpose flour blend

⅓ cup packed light brown sugar

½ teaspoon baking powder

½ teaspoon ground cinnamon

¼ teaspoon fine salt

½ cup (8 tablespoons) unsalted butter, softened to room temperature (use coconut oil or vegan butter, for dairy-free and vegan)

½ teaspoon pure vanilla extract

FOR THE FILLING

2½ cups fresh blueberries

½ cup juice-sweetened blueberry jam or spread

2 teaspoons grated lemon zest (1 lemon)

1 tablespoon fresh lemon juice (from the zested lemon)

½ teaspoon pure vanilla extract

Pinch of fine salt

Lemony, sweet blueberries sandwiched between a buttery oat crust and crumb topping? Yes, please! As their name implies, these bars are like jammy little fruit pies you can hold in your hand (or better yet, one in each hand). They're the perfect way to add a little sweetness to your day.

Preheat the oven to 375°F. Line an 8×8-inch baking pan with parchment paper, leaving 2 inches of overhang on two opposing sides.

Make the crust and topping: Add the oats, flour, brown sugar, baking powder, cinnamon, and salt to a medium bowl and stir to combine. Add the butter and vanilla. Using a large spoon or your hands, work the butter into the oat mixture until you get a crumbly dough that will stick together when you pinch it between your fingers.

Measure 1½ cups of the oat mixture into a small bowl and chill in the refrigerator, for the crumb topping.

Using the back of a spoon, a rubber spatula, or slightly damp fingers, firmly press the remaining oat mixture into the bottom of the prepared baking pan to form the crust. Then use a fork to pierce the crust 8 to 10 times.

Bake the crust for 10 to 12 minutes, or until the edges are just slightly brown and the crust starts to puff and look set.

While the crust is baking, make the filling: Wipe out the medium bowl you used and add the blueberries, blueberry jam, lemon zest, lemon juice, vanilla, and salt and stir to combine.

Spread the filling in an even layer over the hot crust. Crumble the chilled topping over the filling.

Bake for 30 to 35 minutes, or until the topping is lightly browned and the filling is bubbling.

Continued on the next page

Allow to cool completely in the pan on a wire rack, then refrigerate for at least 2 hours before cutting into bars.

To cut the cooled bars, use the parchment paper handles to lift the bars onto a cutting board, then cut into 16 squares.

Store leftovers in an airtight container in the refrigerator for up to 4 days.

Tips from the Dietitians

While it's tempting to the cut into the bars before they have fully cooled, resist the urge to do so. The bars will hold their shape and have a perfectly jamlike filling after they've been chilled. It's worth the wait, we promise!

Nutrition Info: (Serving size: 1 bar) 160 calories, 7g total fat, 4g saturated fat, 65mg sodium, 24g carbs, 9g sugar, 2g fiber, 2g protein

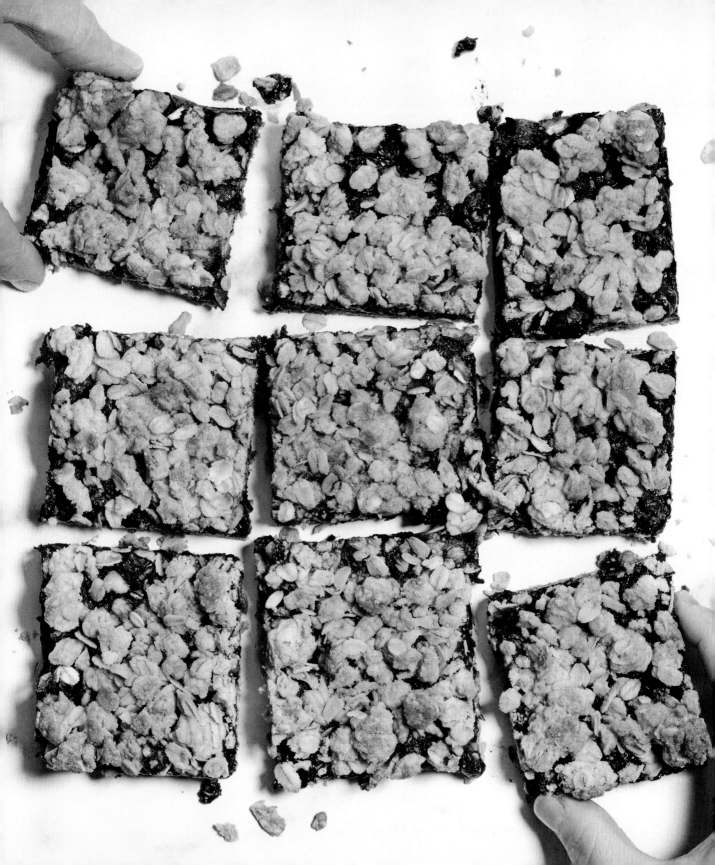

apple cobbler

Prep Time: **30 minutes** | Cook Time: **55 minutes** | Total Time: **1 hour 25 minutes, plus 15 minutes for cooling** | Makes **12 servings**

FOR THE APPLE FILLING

Unsalted butter (or nonstick cooking spray, for dairy-free and vegan), for greasing
5 pounds Granny Smith apples, peeled and sliced into ¼- to ½-inch-thick wedges (12 to 13 cups; see Tips)
½ cup packed light brown sugar
3 tablespoons fresh lemon juice (1 medium lemon)
2 tablespoons gluten-free all-purpose flour blend (or 1 tablespoon cornstarch)
2 teaspoons ground cinnamon
¼ teaspoon ground ginger
Pinch of ground nutmeg
Pinch of fine salt

FOR THE BISCUIT TOPPING

1 cup milk (or nondairy milk, for dairy-free and vegan)
1 teaspoon apple cider vinegar or white vinegar
1 teaspoon pure vanilla extract
2 cups gluten-free all-purpose flour blend
⅓ cup plus 1½ teaspoons granulated sugar, divided
2 teaspoons baking powder
¼ teaspoon baking soda
¼ teaspoon fine salt
6 tablespoons unsalted butter, chilled and cut into small cubes (use vegan butter, for dairy-free and vegan)
¼ teaspoon ground cinnamon

Sweet-tart apples tossed in cinnamon and brown sugar then topped with fluffy, lightly sweetened biscuits give this cobbler all the cozy fall vibes! We grew up in Minnesota and visits to the local apple orchard were a yearly family tradition for both of us, so we knew that this cookbook would not be complete without the perfect fall dessert. Mission accomplished.

Preheat the oven to 350°F. Grease a 9×13-inch baking dish with butter and set aside.

Make the filling: In a large bowl, combine the apples, brown sugar, lemon juice, flour, cinnamon, ginger, nutmeg, and salt. Toss well to combine, then spread the apple mixture into the bottom of the prepared baking dish.

Make the biscuit topping: In a liquid measuring cup, combine the milk, vinegar, and vanilla, and stir. Let stand for 5 minutes.

Meanwhile, in a medium bowl, combine the flour, ⅓ cup granulated sugar, baking powder, baking soda, and salt and stir or whisk. Add the chilled butter. Using a pastry cutter or a fork, cut the butter into the flour until the mixture resembles coarse crumbs. Add the milk mixture to the bowl and stir until a wet dough forms.

Using a spoon, scoop the biscuit topping onto the apples, forming 12 mounds. Use damp fingers to press each mound into a 2-inch disk.

In a small bowl, combine the cinnamon with the remaining 1½ teaspoons granulated sugar and stir. Sprinkle the cinnamon sugar over the biscuit dough.

Bake for 45 to 55 minutes, or until the filling starts to bubble, the apples are tender, and a toothpick inserted into the center of a biscuit comes out clean.

Optional toppings:
Vanilla ice cream, whipped cream, or nondairy whipped topping (for dairy-free and vegan)

Allow to cool for 15 minutes in the pan on a wire rack.

Serve the cobbler warm with your desired topping.

Store leftovers in an airtight container at room temperature for up to 3 days.

Tips from the Dietitians

While we like the tartness of Granny Smith apples for this dessert, you can swap in other varieties that are well-suited for baking, such as Jonagold, Braeburn, or Honeycrisp.

Nutrition Info: (Serving size: $\frac{1}{12}$ of recipe) 220 calories, 7g total fat, 4g saturated fat, 170mg sodium, 28g carbs, 25g sugar, 5g fiber, 2g protein

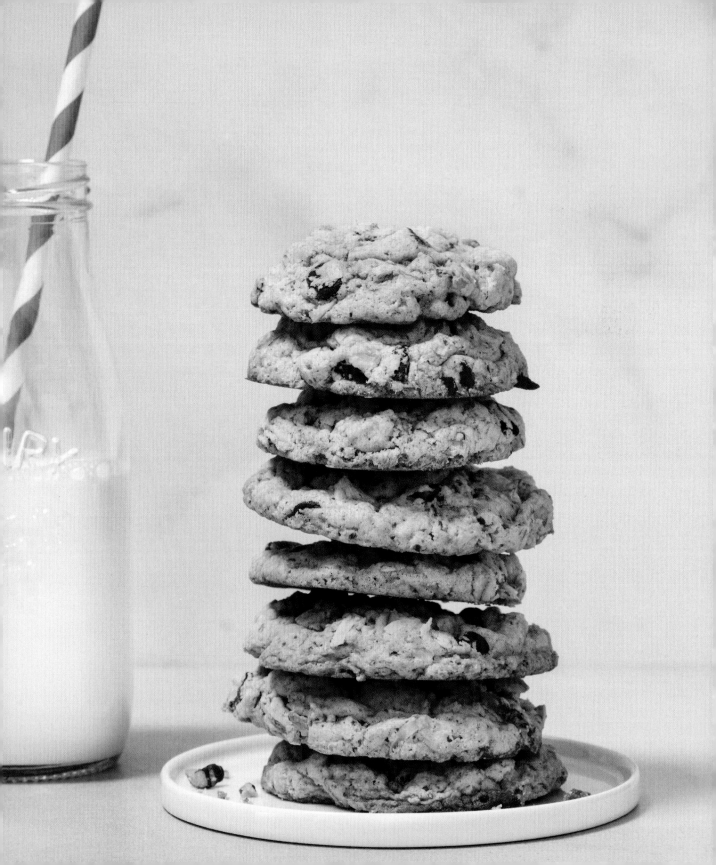

cowgirl cookies

Prep Time: **15 minutes** | Cook Time: **10 minutes** | Total Time: **25 minutes, plus 15 minutes for cooling** | Makes **18 cookies**

GF
DFO
EF
VEG
VO
NFO

1 tablespoon ground flaxseed (see Tips)

3 tablespoons water

⅔ cup packed light brown sugar

½ cup (8 tablespoons) unsalted butter, softened to room temperature (use coconut oil or vegan butter, for dairy-free and vegan)

2 teaspoons pure vanilla extract

1 cup gluten-free all-purpose flour blend

½ teaspoon baking powder

¼ teaspoon baking soda

¼ teaspoon fine salt

½ cup old-fashioned rolled oats

½ cup chocolate chips (use a dairy-free version for dairy-free and vegan)

⅓ cup gluten-free crispy rice cereal

⅓ cup unsweetened shredded coconut

¼ cup chopped pecans (omit for nut-free)

When Jessica was growing up, her dad would make his take on cowboy cookies that he called "Barbara Bush cookies" (the recipe was based on one from Laura Bush, but he could never remember her name, so he attributed them to her mother-in-law). They were chewy chocolate chip cookies with oatmeal, sweetened shredded coconut, and plenty of pecans, and he baked them so often he can still recall the recipe from memory. The cookies here are an egg-free version of those Barbara Bush cookies and every bit as scrumptious. We've reduced the sugar and added crispy rice cereal, which gives a little more crunch along with the nuts.

Position racks in the upper and lower thirds of the oven, and preheat it to 375°F. Line two baking sheets with parchment paper and set aside.

In a small bowl, combine the flaxseed with the water and stir well. Set aside until thickened, 5 to 10 minutes.

Add the brown sugar and butter to a medium bowl (or the bowl of a stand mixer fitted with the flat beater attachment). Using a hand mixer (or the stand mixer), cream the butter and sugar at medium-high speed, scraping down the sides of the bowl as needed, until the mixture is light in color, about 1 minute. Add the flaxseed mixture and vanilla to the bowl. Mix on medium-high speed until the mixture is light and fluffy, 1 to 2 minutes.

In another medium bowl, combine the flour, baking powder, baking soda, and salt. Mix with a fork to combine, then add to the butter mixture and mix on low speed until all of the flour is incorporated. Add the oats, chocolate chips, cereal, coconut, and pecans to the dough, and fold in with a rubber spatula or large spoon.

Using a cookie scoop or spoon, scoop the dough onto the prepared baking sheets, forming 18 mounds.

Continued on the next page

Bake on the upper and lower oven racks for 9 to 11 minutes, rotating and switching the positions of the baking sheets halfway through, or until the cookies are set and the bottoms are lightly browned.

Remove from the oven and allow the cookies to cool on the baking sheets for 5 minutes, then transfer them to a wire rack to cool completely.

Store leftovers in an airtight container at room temperature for up to 4 days or in the freezer for up to 2 months.

Tips from the Dietitians
To make these cookies with an egg, use 1 large egg in place of the ground flaxseed and water.

Nutrition Info: (Serving size: 1 cookie) 146 calories, 9g total fat, 4g saturated fat, 82mg sodium, 16g carbs, 10g sugar, 2g fiber, 2g protein

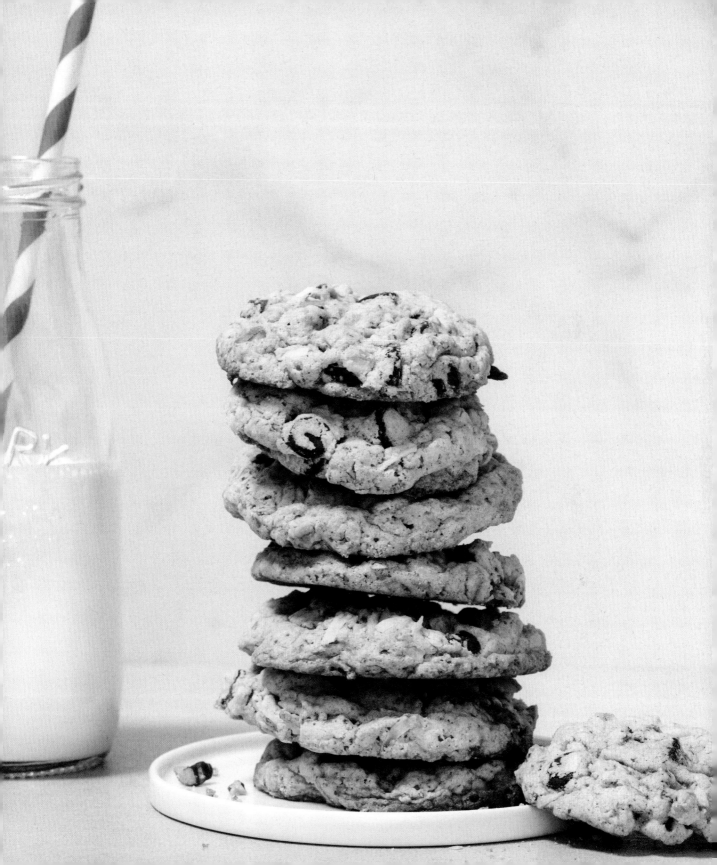

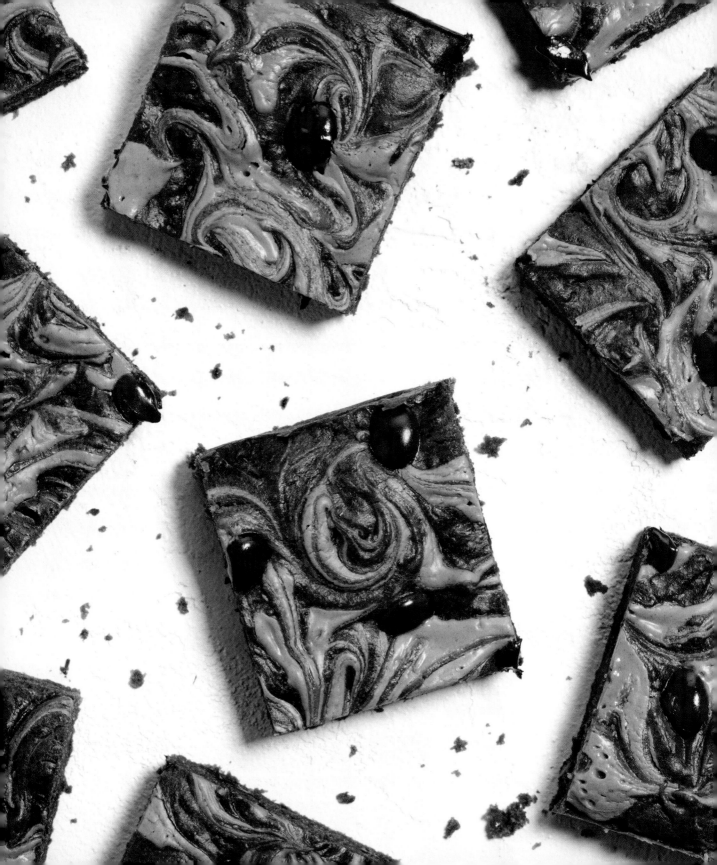

peanut butter swirl brownies

Prep Time: **10 minutes** | Cook Time: **20 minutes** | Total Time: **30 minutes, plus 10 minutes for cooling** | Makes **16 brownies**

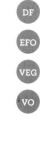

FOR THE BROWNIES
Nonstick cooking spray
⅔ cup gluten-free all-purpose flour blend
¼ cup unsweetened cocoa powder
½ teaspoon baking powder
¼ teaspoon fine salt
½ cup packed light brown sugar
1 large egg (use a flax egg, for vegan and egg-free; see Tips)
1 teaspoon pure vanilla extract
¾ cup natural creamy peanut butter
¾ cup plus 2 tablespoons milk (or nondairy milk, for dairy-free and vegan)
½ cup semisweet or dark chocolate chips (use a dairy-free version for dairy-free and vegan)

FOR THE TOPPING
2 tablespoons creamy natural peanut butter
3 tablespoons semisweet or dark chocolate chips (use a dairy-free version for vegan)

Tips from the Dietitians
To make a flax egg, stir 1 tablespoon of ground flaxseed into 3 tablespoons of water in a small bowl until well combined and let stand for 5 minutes. Use it in place of the 1 large egg in the recipe.

For as long as Stacie can remember, the combination of peanut butter and chocolate has been a favorite of hers. She combines the ever-popular sweet and salty duo in these irresistibly fudgy brownies. For a truly decadent treat worthy of birthday celebrations and anniversaries, serve the brownie warm with a scoop of vanilla ice cream.

Preheat the oven to 350°F. Spray an 8x8-inch baking pan with cooking spray and set aside.

For the brownies: In a large bowl, combine the flour, cocoa powder, baking powder, and salt. Stir and then set aside.

In a medium bowl, combine the brown sugar, egg, and vanilla. Whisk well, then stir in the peanut butter. Add the peanut butter mixture to the bowl with the dry ingredients. Add the milk and stir until just combined, then fold in the chocolate chips.

Transfer the batter to the prepared pan and spread out evenly with a rubber spatula.

For the topping: Dollop or drizzle the peanut butter all over the top of the brownie batter. Using a butter knife, swirl the peanut butter into the brownie batter. Lightly press the chocolate chips into the top of the dough.

Bake for 18 to 20 minutes, or until a toothpick inserted into the center comes out clean. Allow the brownies to cool in the pan on a wire rack for 10 minutes, then cut into 16 squares.

Store leftovers in an airtight container in the refrigerator for up to 1 week or in the freezer for up to 2 months.

Nutrition Info: (Serving size: 1 brownie) 178 calories, 11g total fat, 3g saturated fat, 91mg sodium, 18g carbs, 13g sugar, 2g fiber, 5g protein

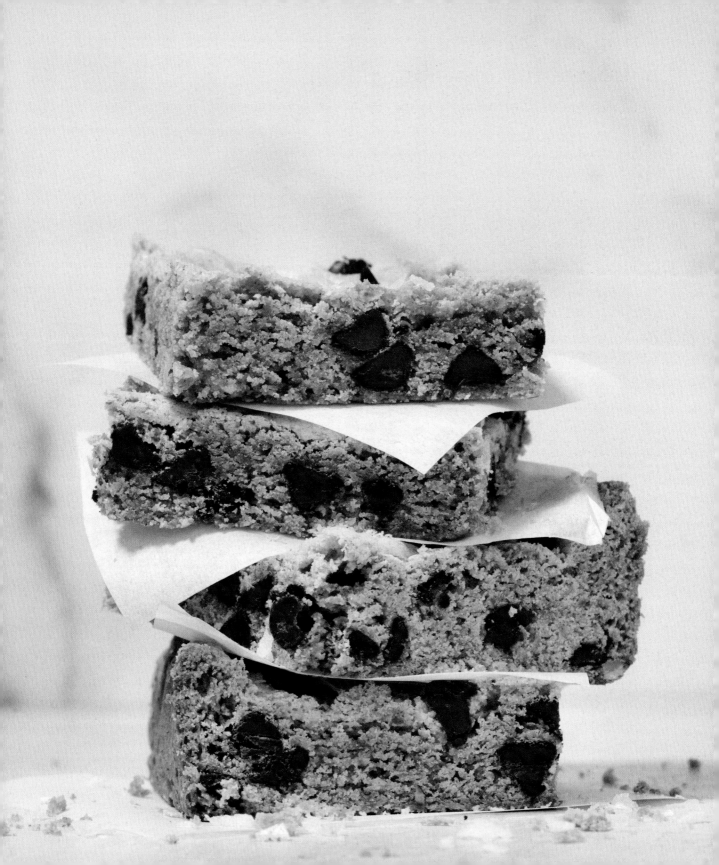

one-bowl chocolate chip blondies

Prep: **15 minutes** | Bake: **30 minutes** | Total: **45 minutes, plus 1 hour for cooling** | Makes **16 blondies**

GF

DFO

EF

VEG

VO

NFO

Nonstick cooking spray

⅔ cup packed light brown sugar

½ cup (8 tablespoons) unsalted butter, softened to room temperature (use coconut oil or vegan butter, for dairy-free and vegan)

3 to 4 tablespoons milk (or nondairy milk, for dairy-free and vegan)

3 tablespoons natural creamy almond butter (use tahini for nut-free)

1 tablespoon pure vanilla extract

1¼ cups gluten-free all-purpose flour blend

¾ teaspoon baking powder

¼ teaspoon fine salt

⅛ teaspoon baking soda

½ cup chocolate chips, plus a few more for pressing into the top of the dough (use a dairy-free version for dairy-free and vegan)

½ teaspoon flaky sea salt (optional)

Tips from the Dietitians

The blondies can also be served warm with a scoop of your favorite ice cream or nondairy frozen dessert for an ooey-gooey treat.

With their buttery, crisp edges and chewy centers, these bars fall somewhere between a cookie and a brownie. A sprinkle of flaky sea salt adds the tiniest bit of salty crunch that perfectly complements the sweetness of the chocolate chips and brown sugar.

Preheat the oven to 350°F. Generously spray an 8x8-inch baking pan with cooking spray and set aside.

In a medium bowl (or the bowl of a stand mixer fitted with the flat beater attachment), combine the brown sugar, butter, 3 tablespoons of the milk, the almond butter, and vanilla. Using a hand mixer (or the stand mixer), beat at medium-high speed until the mixture is smooth and fluffy, about 2 minutes.

Add the flour, baking powder, fine salt, and baking soda to the bowl and slowly beat at medium speed until combined and a very soft dough forms, about 1 minute. If the dough is dry or very stiff, beat in an additional 1 tablespoon of milk. Using a rubber spatula or large spoon, fold the ½ cup chocolate chips into the dough.

Spread the dough evenly into the prepared baking pan. Lightly press the extra chocolate chips into the top of the dough.

Bake for 24 to 27 minutes, or until the edges are golden brown, the center is set, and a toothpick inserted in the center comes out clean.

Remove the pan from the oven and sprinkle the blondies with the flaky sea salt, if using.

Allow the blondies to cool completely in the pan on a wire rack, then slice into 16 squares.

Store leftovers in an airtight container at room temperature for up to 4 days or in the freezer for up to 2 months.

Nutrition Info: (Serving size: 1 blondie without the optional ingredients) 175 calories, 9g total fat, 5g saturated fat, 79mg sodium, 22g carbs, 13g sugar, 2g fiber, 2g protein

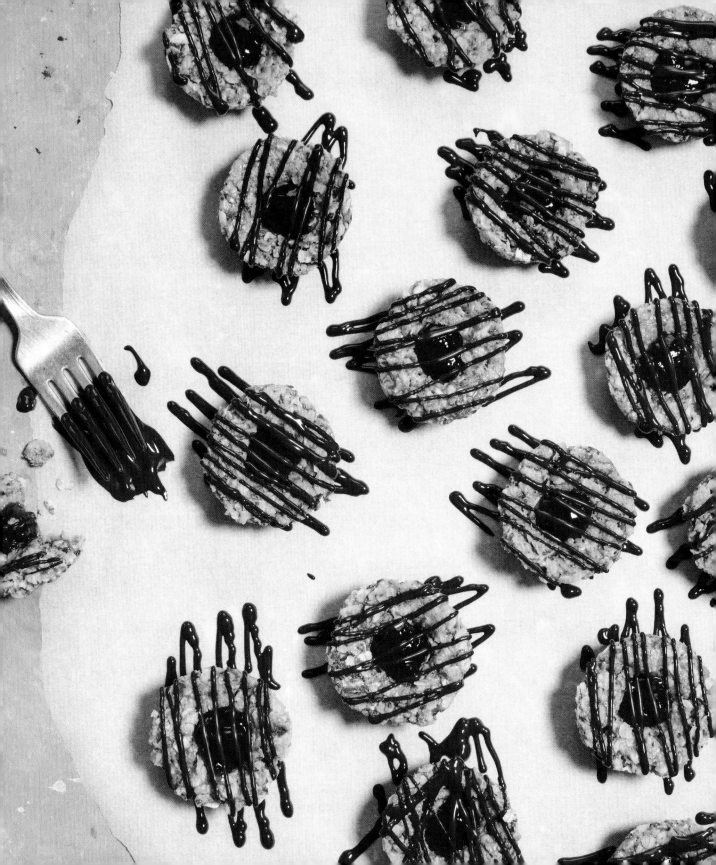

no-bake peanut butter & jelly crunch bites

Prep Time: **25 minutes** | Total Time: **25 minutes** | Makes **32 bites (16 servings)**

2 cups quick-cooking oats

1 cup gluten-free crispy rice cereal

⅓ cup unsweetened shredded coconut

⅓ cup ground flaxseed

1 tablespoon chia seeds

1 cup plus 2 tablespoons natural creamy peanut butter

⅓ cup honey

2 tablespoons coconut oil, melted, plus 1 teaspoon for the chocolate

1½ teaspoons pure vanilla extract

1 to 2 tablespoons water

3 tablespoons juice-sweetened strawberry jam or spread

¼ cup chocolate chips (use a dairy-free version for dairy-free)

Tips from the Dietitians

A silicone mini muffin pan makes it especially easy to remove the bites.

To create this sweet treat, we adapted our recipe for Peanut Butter Crunch Bars from the blog to include the cutest little dollop of strawberry preserves on each bite, then drizzled them with melted chocolate for a slightly more grown-up version of a childhood favorite.

In a medium bowl, combine the oats, cereal, coconut, flaxseed, and chia seeds. Stir to combine.

Add the peanut butter, honey, 2 tablespoons of the coconut oil, and vanilla to the bowl and mix well. The dough should stick together easily, if not, add water, 1 tablespoon at a time, until the dough sticks together when pressed between your fingers.

Using a spoon, divide the mixture evenly among 32 mini muffin cups (depending on the size of your pan, you may need more than one; see Tips). Press the mixture very firmly into each cup. Using your finger or the end of a wooden spoon, create an indentation in the center of each bite. Fill each with ¼ teaspoon of the jam.

Place the muffin pan(s) in the freezer for about 20 minutes, or until the bites are very firm.

Just before removing the bites from the freezer, in a small saucepan over low heat, combine the chocolate chips and remaining 1 teaspoon coconut oil. Cook, stirring occasionally, until the chocolate is smooth, 2 to 3 minutes.

Remove the muffin pan(s) from the freezer and transfer the bites to a parchment-lined baking sheet. If not using silicone mini muffin pan(s), slide a knife between each bite and the cup then gently lift up to remove. Drizzle each bite with the melted chocolate.

Store leftovers in the refrigerator for up to 1 week or in the freezer for up to 4 months.

Nutrition Info: (Serving size: 2 bites) 247 calories, 14g total fat, 4g saturated fat, 45mg sodium, 23g carbs, 9g sugar, 4g fiber, 7g protein

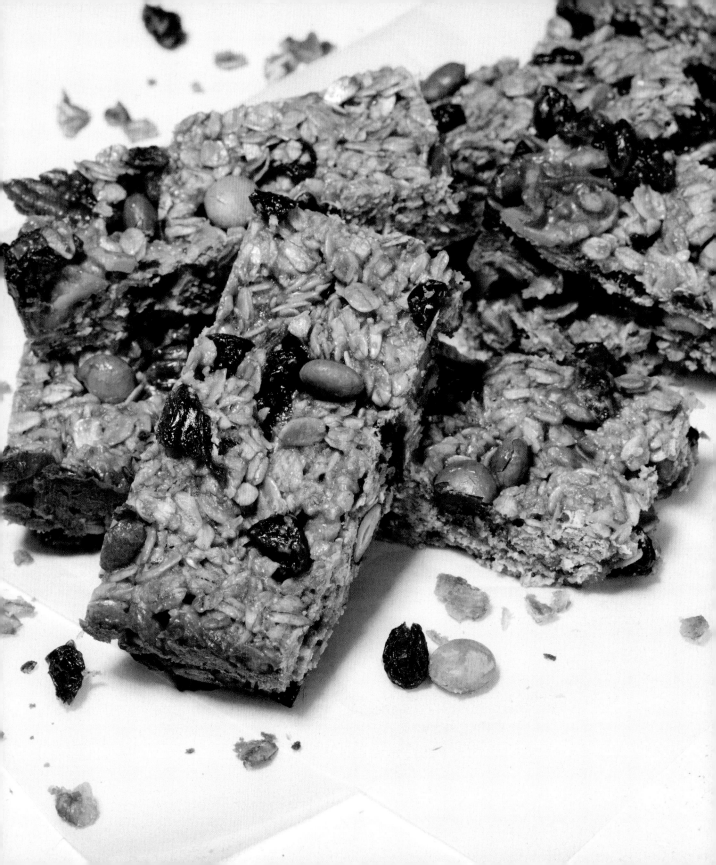

trail mix granola bars

Prep Time: **10 minutes** | Cook Time: **30 minutes** | Total Time: **40 minutes, plus 1 hour for cooling** | Makes **12 bars**

GF

DFO

VEG

2½ cups old-fashioned rolled oats

2 large eggs

½ cup natural creamy peanut butter

⅓ cup honey

2 tablespoons avocado oil or extra-virgin olive oil

1½ teaspoons pure vanilla extract

1½ cups packaged trail mix of choice (or substitute mixed nuts, seeds, and/or dried fruits of choice)

Whether you're running errands with kids, planning a big hike, or need a little something to add to a lunch box or backpack, these chewy granola bars will quickly become your go-to snack. They're simple to make, and you call the shots when it comes to the type of packaged trail mix to add, so they're easy to customize to suit your taste (and cravings).

Preheat the oven to 325°F. Line an 8×8-inch baking pan with parchment paper, leaving 2 inches of overhang on two opposing sides, and set aside.

In a medium bowl, combine the oats, eggs, peanut butter, honey, avocado oil, and vanilla. Stir to combine, then fold in the trail mix.

Using a rubber spatula, firmly press the oat mixture into the prepared baking pan in an even layer.

Bake for 25 to 27 minutes, or until the middle is set and the edges and bottom are light golden brown (use the parchment paper to gently lift a corner of the bars to see the bottom).

Remove from the oven and allow the bars to cool in the pan on a wire rack for 5 minutes.

Use the parchment paper handles to lift the bars onto a wire rack to cool completely, then slice into 12 bars or squares.

Store leftovers in an airtight container in the refrigerator for up to 1 week or in the freezer for up to 2 months.

Tips from the Dietitians

If you're looking for a vegan sweet snack to pack on your next adventure, try our No-Bake Energy Bites Three Ways (page 248) and swap the chocolate chips in that recipe for your favorite trail mix.

Nutrition Info: (Serving size: 1 bar) 280 calories, 15g total fat, 2g saturated fat, 39mg sodium, 31g carbs, 12g sugar, 4g fiber, 6g protein

no-bake energy bites three ways

Prep Time: **25 minutes** | Total Time: **25 minutes** | Makes **22 to 24 bites**

GF
DFO
VEG
VO

1½ cups old-fashioned rolled oats, plus more if the dough is too wet

3 tablespoons ground flaxseed

1 tablespoon chia seeds

Pinch of fine salt

¾ cup natural creamy nut butter (choose the one for Coconut-Almond, Peanut Butter Chocolate Chip, or Oatmeal Raisin; options follow)

¼ cup pure maple syrup

1 teaspoon pure vanilla extract

¼ teaspoon pure almond extract (for Coconut-Almond)

Mix-ins (choose the ones for Coconut-Almond, Peanut Butter Chocolate Chip, or Oatmeal Raisin; options follow)

For these easy, energy-packed snacks, we took the same oat-and-seed base and changed up the type of nut butter and mix-ins to create three flavors: coconut-almond, peanut butter chocolate chip, and oatmeal raisin (or cranberry). Nut butters can vary in consistency from brand to brand (and even by type of nut), so the one you use may affect the outcome of your dough. If your dough is too dry to roll into balls, mix in more water; too wet, add more oats. The energy bites freeze well, so they're great to make ahead and have on hand for an afternoon treat or preworkout snack whenever you need one.

If you prefer to make the energy bites with a chunkier texture, skip to the next step. This optional step helps to achieve a smoother texture in the energy bites. Add the oats to a food processor or blender. Pulse until some of the oats are broken into very small pieces and others remain relatively intact, 10 to 15 times.

In a medium bowl, combine the oats, flaxseed, chia seeds, salt, nut butter, maple syrup, vanilla, and almond extract (for Coconut-Almond). Stir with a wooden spoon or mix with clean hands until well combined. Add the mix-ins for your chosen flavor and stir. Refrigerate for 15 minutes.

Using your hands, roll the chilled dough into 22 to 24 balls, each about 1½ tablespoons. If the dough is too dry for a ball to hold its shape, add 1 tablespoon of water at a time to the dough and stir until it sticks together easily. If the dough is too wet, add 1 tablespoon of oats at a time. If the dough sticks to your hands when rolling it into balls, coat your hands with a few drops of water to prevent sticking.

Store in an airtight container in the refrigerator for up to 2 weeks or in the freezer for up to 2 months.

coconut almond energy bites

GF
DFO
VEG
VO

¾ cup natural creamy almond
butter (see Tips)

MIX-INS:
3 tablespoons mini chocolate
chips or roughly chopped
regular chocolate chips (use a
dairy-free version, for dairy-free
and vegan)
2 tablespoons unsweetened
shredded coconut
2 tablespoons chopped dry
roasted almonds

Tips from the Dietitians
Natural almond butter with a smooth and runny consistency works best
in this recipe.

Nutrition Info: (Serving size: 1 bite) 105 calories, 6g total fat, 1g saturated fat, 25mg sodium,
10g carbs, 4g sugar, 2g fiber, 3g protein

peanut butter chocolate chip energy bites

GF
DFO
VEG
VO

¾ cup natural creamy peanut
butter (see Tips)

MIX-INS:
⅓ cup mini chocolate chips
or roughly chopped regular
chocolate chips (use a dairy-
free version for dairy-free and
vegan)

Tips from the Dietitians
It's best to use peanut butter that has a runny (almost drizzly)
consistency. If the peanut butter is too thick at room temperature,
simply heat it slightly in the microwave for 10 to 20 seconds, then stir to
achieve a thinner consistency.

Nutrition Info: (Serving size: 1 bite) 103 calories, 6g total fat, 1g saturated fat, 27mg sodium,
11g carbs, 4g sugar, 2g fiber, 3g protein

Continued on the next page

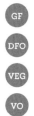

oatmeal raisin or cranberry energy bites

¾ cup natural creamy cashew
   butter

MIX-INS:

⅓ cup dark raisins or dried
   cranberries

Tips from the Dietitians

It's best to use cashew butter that has a very smooth consistency that isn't too thick. If the cashew butter is too thick at room temperature, simply heat it slightly in the microwave for 10 to 20 seconds, then stir to achieve a thinner consistency.

Nutrition Info: (Serving size: 1 bite) 89 calories, 5g total fat, 1g saturated fat, 9mg sodium, 10g carbs, 2g sugar, 2g fiber, 3g protein

easy fruit dip two ways

Prep Time: **5 minutes** | Total Time: **5 minutes** | Makes **4 servings**

1 cup plain Greek yogurt
1 teaspoon pure vanilla extract
Peanut Butter Flavor or Pumpkin
   Pie Flavor (options follow)

PEANUT BUTTER FLAVOR

⅓ cup natural creamy peanut
   butter
2 tablespoons honey
¼ teaspoon ground cinnamon

Optional toppings:
Chopped peanuts and a dusting
   of ground cinnamon

PUMPKIN PIE FLAVOR

⅓ cup pumpkin puree
2 tablespoons pure maple syrup
¼ teaspoon pumpkin pie spice

Optional toppings:
Chopped pecans (omit for nut-
   free) and a dusting of pumpkin
   pie spice
Fruit, pretzels, and/or graham
   crackers (gluten-free, if desired),
   for dipping

Fruit by itself is delicious, but when dunked into one of these fruit dips it becomes an extra special and fun after-school snack or healthy dessert. Our dips have just enough natural sweetener to satisfy a sweet craving without ruining your dinner when enjoyed as an afternoon snack. They can also be served at birthday parties, baby showers, and any other special occasions as part of a better-for-you spread. Choose from two flavors to mix into the Greek yogurt base: peanut butter or pumpkin pie. Serve the dip with your choice of fruit, such as strawberries, grapes, sliced apples and bananas, or with pretzels or graham crackers.

In a small bowl, combine the yogurt and vanilla with the ingredients for either the peanut butter or pumpkin pie flavor and stir to mix well.

Serve with your desired toppings and fruit, pretzels, and/or graham crackers. Store leftovers in an airtight container in the refrigerator for up to 4 days.

For Peanut Butter Flavor
Nutrition Info: (Serving size: ⅓ cup without the optional toppings and accompaniments) 201 calories, 12g total fat, 2g saturated fat, 65mg sodium, 16g carbs, 12g sugar, 1g fiber, 10g protein

For Pumpkin Pie Flavor
Nutrition Info: (Serving size: ⅓ cup without the optional toppings) 78 calories, 1g total fat, 1g saturated fat, 21mg sodium, 11g carbs, 9g sugar, 1g fiber, 6g protein

condiments & sauces

Dairy-Free Ranch Dressing & Dip

Ranch Seasoning Mix

Greek Vinaigrette & Marinade

Honey Mustard Dressing & Dipping Sauce

Homemade Barbecue Sauce

Peanut Dressing & Dipping Sauce

Six-Ingredient Pico de Gallo

Quick-Pickled Onions

Quick-Pickled Carrots or Cucumbers

Garlic-Herb Croutons

dairy-free ranch dressing & dip

GF GrF DF EFO VEG VO NF

Prep Time: **5 minutes** | Total Time: **5 minutes** | Makes **1 cup (8 servings)**

½ cup mayonnaise (or vegan mayonnaise, for egg-free and vegan; see Tips)

¼ cup full-fat canned coconut milk (see Tips)

2 tablespoons Ranch Seasoning Mix, plus more as needed

1 tablespoon apple cider vinegar

Fine salt and ground black pepper

Creamy, flavorful, and made with ingredients you can pronounce, this dressing features a dairy-free base mixed with our homemade Ranch Seasoning Mix (page 257). Stacie always has a jar in her refrigerator for dressing salads, dipping vegetables, making Bacon Ranch Deviled Eggs (page 211), or drizzling over Ranch Roasted Potatoes (page 61) or Buffalo Chicken–Stuffed Spaghetti Squash (page 81). Don't be surprised if you never buy another bottle of premade ranch dressing again.

In a small bowl, combine the mayonnaise, coconut milk, Ranch Seasoning Mix, and vinegar and stir to mix well. Add salt and pepper and more Ranch Seasoning Mix to taste.

Cover and refrigerate until ready to serve. Store in an airtight container or mason jar in the refrigerator for up to 1 week.

Tips from the Dietitians

If the liquid is separated from the solid fat inside the can of coconut milk, blend them in a blender until smooth. Store any unused coconut milk in an airtight container for up to 4 days.

If you don't need this recipe to be dairy-free, you can substitute plain yogurt, sour cream, or buttermilk for the coconut milk.

For a thinner consistency, add 1 to 2 tablespoons of your milk of choice (use nondairy milk for dairy-free and vegan).

If you're looking to avoid added sugars, use mayonnaise that is made without sugar.

Nutrition Info: (Serving size: 2 tablespoons) 108 calories, 11g total fat, 3g saturated fat, 165mg sodium, 1g carbs, 0g sugar, 0g fiber, 0g protein

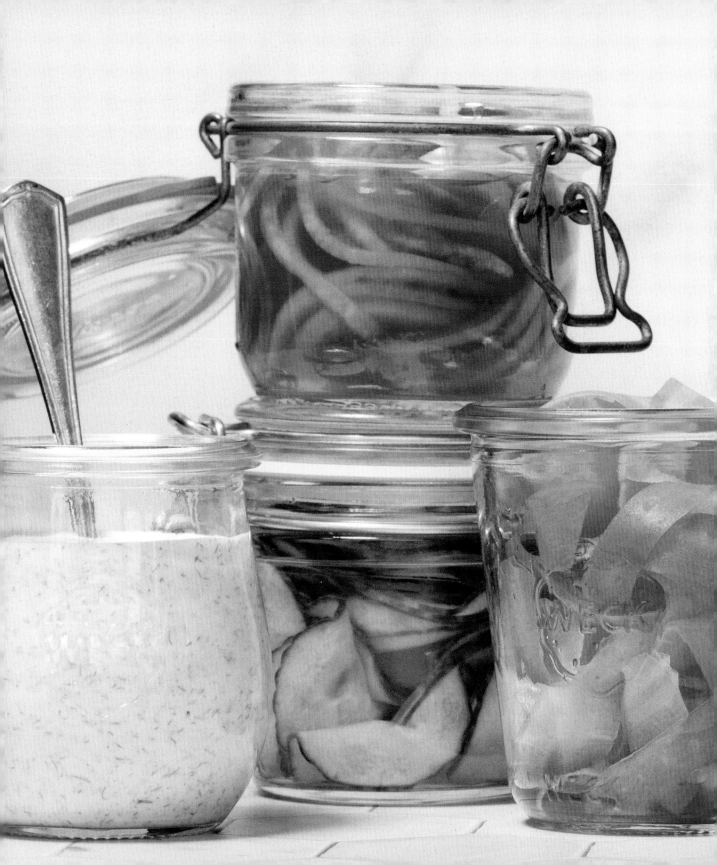

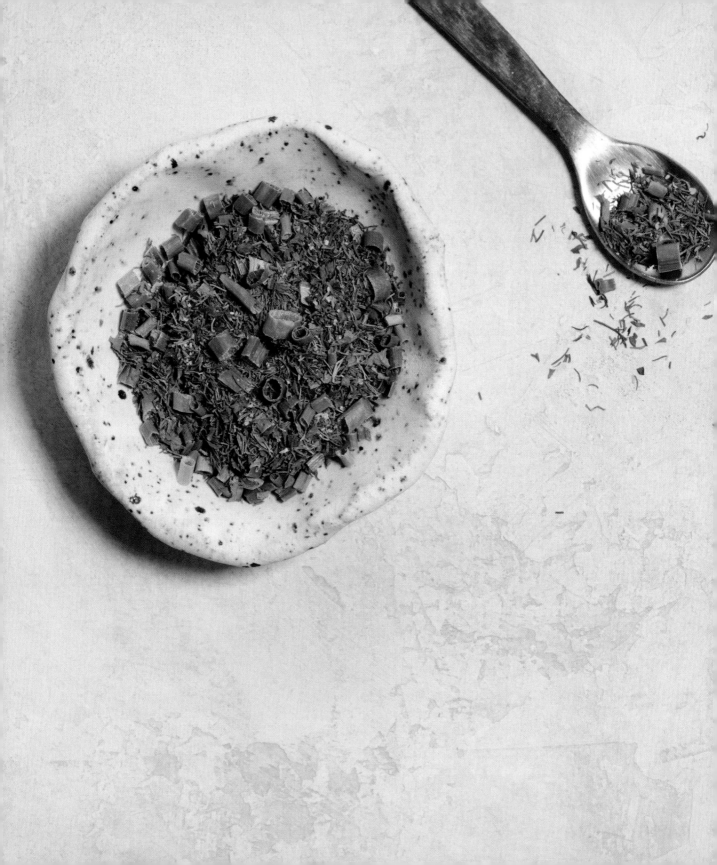

ranch seasoning mix

Prep Time: **5 minutes** | Total Time: **5 minutes** | Makes **½ cup**

¼ cup dried dill
2 tablespoons dried parsley
2 tablespoons dried chives
1 tablespoon onion powder
1 tablespoon garlic powder
1 teaspoon fine salt
½ teaspoon ground black pepper

Skip the packet and make your own! Not only is our homemade ranch seasoning budget friendly, it's free of preservatives, sugar, and artificial flavors. We like to keep it on hand to quickly whip up a batch of salad dressing, add to any dish that could use a little extra flavor, or use it to season meat, eggs, or vegetables (see Tips). It's also delicious sprinkled on buttered popcorn.

In a bowl or mason jar, combine the dill, parsley, chives, onion powder, garlic powder, salt, and pepper and stir well.

Store in an airtight container at room temperature for up to 1 year.

Tips from the Dietitians
Use this Ranch Seasoning Mix for the quickest and easiest Dairy-Free Ranch Dressing and Dip (page 254), Ranch Roasted Potatoes (page 61), or Ranch Party Mix (page 199).

GF
GrF
DF
EF
V
NF
NAS

Nutrition Info: (Serving size: 1 teaspoon) 4 calories, 0g total fat, 0g saturated fat, 100mg sodium, 1g carbs, 0g sugar, 0g fiber, 0g protein

greek vinaigrette & marinade

Prep Time: **10 minutes** | Total Time: **10 minutes** | Makes **1 cup (8 servings)**

GF
GrF
DF
EF
V
NF
NAS

⅔ cup avocado oil or extra-virgin olive oil

¼ cup red wine vinegar

¼ cup fresh lemon juice (1 large lemon)

2 garlic cloves, grated or finely minced

1 teaspoon dried oregano

1 teaspoon fine salt

½ teaspoon ground black pepper

You'll be amazed at how much flavor this vinaigrette can add to a simple garden salad, pasta salad, or meals, like our Greek Chicken Meatball Bowls with Tzatziki (page 103). We've kept this recipe dairy-free so it can be used as a marinade for meat, seafood, or vegetables. If you're craving a creamy dressing, be sure to check out our Greek Chopped Salad (page 49), where we add Greek yogurt and feta to this vinaigrette.

Add the avocado oil, vinegar, lemon juice, garlic, oregano, salt, and pepper to a small bowl and whisk to combine. Alternatively, add all of the ingredients to a jar with a tight-fitting lid and shake well to combine.

Use as desired, or store in an airtight container in the refrigerator for up to 1 week.

If the oil in the dressing has solidified in the refrigerator, let the dressing stand at room temperature (or run the container under warm water) until liquid again, then shake well before using.

Tips from the Dietitians
To use this vinaigrette as a marinade: Combine 1 pound of meat (thawed, if frozen) with ½ cup of the vinaigrette in a zip-top bag or airtight container, and marinate in the refrigerator for 30 minutes to 4 hours before cooking.

Nutrition Info: (Serving size: 2 tablespoons) 166 calories, 18g total fat, 2g saturated fat, 295mg sodium, 1g carbs, 0g sugar, 0g fiber, 0g protein

honey mustard dressing & dipping sauce

Prep Time: **10 minutes** | Total Time: **10 minutes** | Makes ¾ cup **(6 servings)**

½ cup mayonnaise (or vegan mayonnaise, for egg-free)

¼ cup spicy brown mustard or Dijon mustard

2 tablespoons honey, plus more as needed

¼ teaspoon dried thyme

¼ teaspoon garlic powder

½ teaspoon fine salt, plus more as needed

¼ teaspoon ground black pepper, plus more as needed

We like our honey mustard dressing slightly sweet and tangy, especially on a Big Cobb Salad for Two (page 51) with loads of savory flavors and textures. This recipe also makes a fantastic dip for dunking our Crispy Baked Chicken Nuggets (page 85) or Baked Sweet Potato Fries (see page 65), or for drizzling over grilled chicken or pork chops.

Add the mayonnaise, mustard, honey, thyme, garlic powder, salt, and pepper to a small bowl and whisk to combine. Add more honey, salt, and/or pepper to taste.

Use as desired, or store in an airtight container or mason jar in the refrigerator for up to 1 week.

Nutrition Info: (Serving size: 2 tablespoons) 150 calories, 14g total fat, 2g saturated fat, 410mg sodium, 4g carbs, 4g sugar, 0g fiber, 0g protein

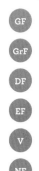

GF

GrF

DF

EF

V

NF

homemade barbecue sauce

Prep Time: **10 minutes** | Cook Time: **40 minutes** | Total Time: **50 minutes** | Makes **2 cups (16 servings)**

1 tablespoon avocado oil or extra-virgin olive oil

½ small yellow onion, diced small (1 cup)

2 garlic cloves, minced

1 (14-ounce) can crushed tomatoes

3 tablespoons apple cider vinegar

2 tablespoons tomato paste

2 tablespoons packed light brown sugar

1 tablespoon molasses

1 tablespoon stone-ground or Dijon mustard

1½ teaspoons smoked paprika

1 teaspoon chili powder

½ teaspoon fine salt, plus more as needed

Most bottled barbecue sauces are loaded with sugar, which makes them taste great, but we're confident this homemade sauce will win you over and help you break the bottle habit. Made with just enough brown sugar and molasses and the perfect amount of spice to complement the natural sweetness of the crushed tomatoes, it's a sauce you'll want to put on everything. We love to pair it with our Instant Pot Pulled Pork (page 155) or Easier-Than-Ever Slow Cooker Baby Back Ribs (page 158) for a meal that rivals one from our favorite barbecue joint. Barbecue sauce can also be brushed onto grilled chicken or pork chops during the last ten minutes of cooking time to add extra flavor. It's also delicious as a dipping sauce for our Crispy Baked Chicken Nuggets (page 85).

Place a medium saucepan over medium-high heat. When hot, add the avocado oil and swirl to coat the bottom. Add the onion and cook, stirring occasionally, until softened and translucent, 7 to 8 minutes. Add the garlic and cook, stirring often, until the garlic is fragrant, about 1 minute.

Add the crushed tomatoes, vinegar, tomato paste, brown sugar, molasses, mustard, paprika, chili powder, and ½ teaspoon salt. Stir well to combine and simmer, stirring occasionally, until thickened, 30 to 35 minutes. Taste, and add more salt, if needed.

Remove from the heat and allow the sauce to cool slightly, then transfer to a blender and blend until smooth.

Use as desired, or store the sauce in an airtight container in the refrigerator for up to 2 weeks.

Tips from the Dietitians
For a smokier flavor, add a few drops of liquid smoke.

Nutrition Info: (Serving size: 2 tablespoons) 33 calories, 1g total fat, 0g saturated fat, 105mg sodium, 5g carbs, 4g sugar, 1g fiber, 1g protein

peanut dressing & dipping sauce

Prep Time: **10 minutes** | Total Time: **10 minutes** | Makes **¾ cup plus 2 tablespoons (7 servings)**

GF
GrF
DF
EF
V
NFO
NAS

⅓ cup natural creamy peanut
   butter
¼ cup coconut aminos
3 tablespoons fresh lime juice
   (1 medium lime)
2 teaspoons rice vinegar
1½ teaspoons toasted sesame oil
1 teaspoon grated peeled
   fresh ginger (1-inch piece; or
   substitute ¼ teaspoon ground
   ginger)
1 garlic clove, minced
½ teaspoon crushed red pepper
   flakes
¼ teaspoon fine salt
Warm water, as needed

Whether you're dressing or dipping, this flavorful and easy-to-make peanut sauce is perfect for serving with Asian-inspired dishes. We use it as a dressing for our quinoa bowls (page 183) and as a dipping sauce for summer rolls (page 215).

In a small bowl, combine the peanut butter, coconut aminos, lime juice, vinegar, sesame oil, ginger, garlic, crushed red pepper flakes, and salt. Whisk until smooth and well combined.

If needed, whisk in warm water 1 teaspoon at a time to achieve a smooth dressinglike consistency. This will depend on the consistency of your peanut butter.

Store any leftover sauce in an airtight container in the refrigerator for up to 4 days.

Tips from the Dietitians
To make the sauce peanut-free, use sunflower seed butter or almond butter in place of the peanut butter.

To make this nut-free, use sunflower seed butter in place of the peanut butter.

Nutrition Info: (Serving size: 2 tablespoons) 91 calories, 7g total fat, 1g saturated fat, 298mg sodium, 5g carbs, 3g sugar, 1g fiber, 3g protein

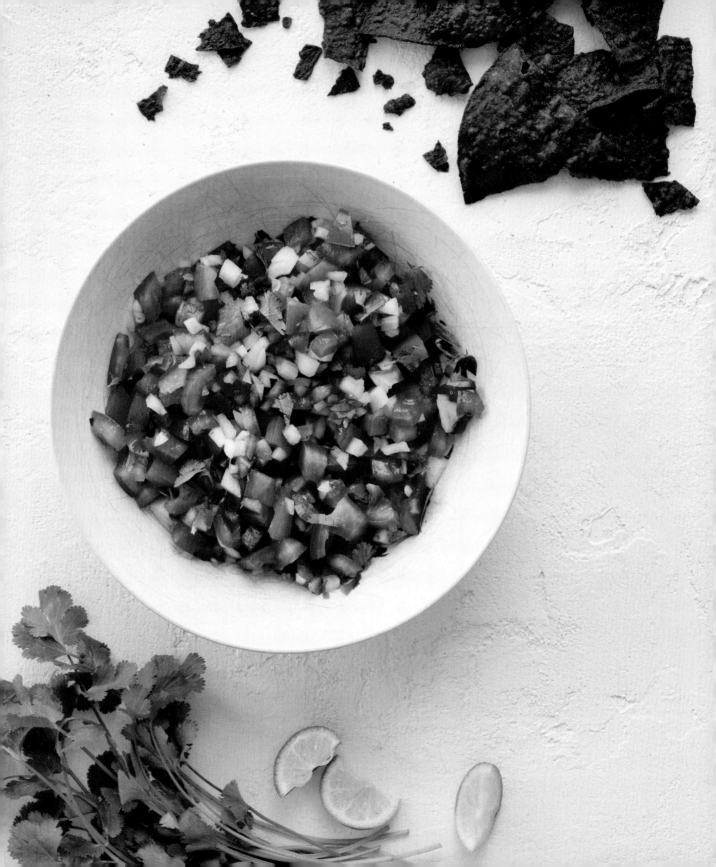

six-ingredient pico de gallo

Prep Time: **20 minutes** | Total Time: **20 minutes** | Makes **3 cups (6 servings)**

GF
GrF
DF
EF
V
NF
NAS

3 Roma tomatoes, quartered, seeded, and diced

½ cup loosely packed fresh cilantro leaves, roughly chopped

½ small white onion, finely chopped

1 small jalapeño, seeds and membranes removed, finely minced (optional; see Tips)

1 garlic clove, grated or finely minced

2 tablespoons fresh lime juice (1 medium lime)

½ teaspoon fine salt

Because Jessica's favorite taco truck never seems to put enough pico de gallo in the bag, she decided to make her own. But when it comes to pico, there are no rules for us—we basically put it on everything. This restaurant-style condiment is, of course, delicious served with tacos or burritos or scooped up with your favorite tortilla chips (see Tips for more serving suggestions). Be sure to bookmark this recipe for summertime when tomatoes are at their best, because every backyard barbecue and gathering benefits from big bowls of pico de gallo and guac, like our Loaded Guacamole (page 203).

Add the tomatoes, cilantro, onion, jalapeño, garlic, lime juice, and salt to a bowl and stir to combine.

Serve as desired. Store leftovers in an airtight container in the refrigerator for up to 3 days.

Tips from the Dietitians

Removing the seeds and membranes from the jalapeño decreases the amount of heat they add to the recipe. Leave them in if you like your pico spicy!

Pico de gallo is a tasty topping for tacos or burrito bowls, like our Fish Tacos with Avocado "Crema" (page 169) and Sweet Potato and Black Bean Burrito Bowls (page 186). You can also dollop the pico on tacos or bowls made with our Instant Pot Beef Barbacoa Burrito Bowls (page 123), Sheet Pan Steak Fajitas (page 127), Turkey Taco Casserole (page 109), or Slow Cooker Tacos al Pastor (page 129). We also like to stir a little pico de gallo into our Dairy-Free Nacho Cheese (page 207).

Nutrition Info: (Serving size: ½ cup without the optional ingredients) 17 calories, 0g total fat, 0g saturated fat, 201mg sodium, 4g carbs, 2g sugar, 1g fiber, 1g protein

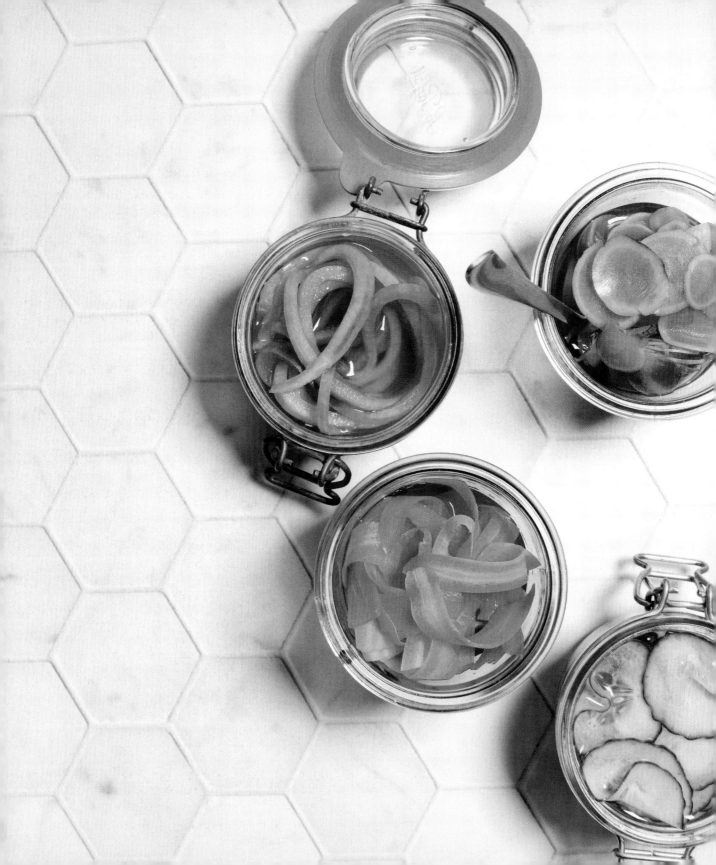

quick-pickled onions

Prep Time: **15 minutes** | Total Time: **15 minutes, plus 1 hour for pickling** | Makes **1½ cups (6 servings)**

GF
GrF
DF
EF
V
NF
NAS

1 cup warm water
1 cup apple cider vinegar
2 teaspoons sugar (omit for no added sugar)
¾ teaspoon fine salt
1 medium red onion, thinly sliced into rings (see Tips)

Pickled onions are a great addition to everything, but they're especially amazing on spicy Mexican-inspired dishes, like tacos and burrito bowls. They add a salty-tangy element that's much like a pickle but different (in a really good way!). We also love to pile these pickled onions atop a juicy burger or a salad, or chop them finely to mix into tuna salad in place of raw onions.

In a wide-mouth quart jar with a lid, combine the water, vinegar, sugar, if using, and salt and stir until the salt and sugar are dissolved. Add the onion to the jar, pressing down to submerge the rings in the liquid.

Cover the jar loosely with the lid and let stand at room temperature for 1 hour before serving.

Store leftovers in the jar, covered, in the refrigerator for up to 2 weeks.

Tips from the Dietitians
You can substitute 6 ounces of trimmed and thinly sliced radishes for the sliced onions.

Nutrition Info: (Serving size: ¼ cup without the optional ingredients) 10 calories, 0g total fat, 0g saturated fat, 49mg sodium, 2g carbs, 1g sugar, 0g fiber, 0g protein

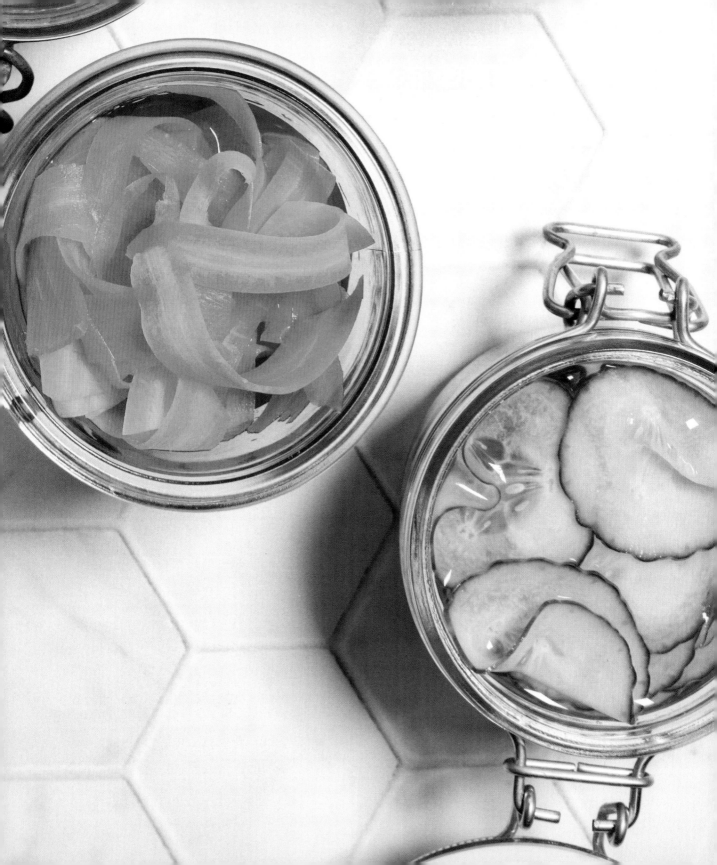

quick-pickled carrots or cucumbers

Prep Time: **15 minutes** | Total Time: **15 minutes, plus 1 hour for pickling** | Makes **3 cups (6 servings)**

GF

GrF

DF

EF

V

NF

NAS

1 cup warm water
1 cup rice vinegar (see Tips)
1 teaspoon sugar (omit for no
    added sugar)
¾ teaspoon fine salt
3 medium carrots, peeled and
    shaved into long ribbons with
    a vegetable peeler, or 1 large
    English cucumber, thinly sliced
    into rounds (about 3 cups)

Jessica makes these tangy pickles at least twice a month because it's one of the ways she can get her daughters to eagerly eat vegetables. She serves them with Asian-inspired dishes, like our Turkey-Mushroom Lettuce Wraps (page 113) or Sticky Teriyaki Chicken Wings (page 209) and a side of Coconut-Lime Rice (page 71). They're also delicious added to salads or served on top of a juicy burger or turkey sandwich, or anywhere you want to add a little tang and crunch.

In a wide-mouth quart jar with a lid, combine the water, vinegar, sugar, if using, and salt and stir until the salt and sugar are dissolved.

Add the carrots to the jar, pressing down to submerge them in the liquid.

Cover the jar loosely with the lid and let stand at room temperature for 1 hour before serving.

Store leftover pickled carrots or cucumbers in the jar, covered, in the refrigerator for up to 1 week.

> **Tips from the Dietitians**
> Don't have rice vinegar? Apple cider vinegar will also work. Just increase the water to 1¼ cups and decrease the vinegar to ¾ cup to account for the more pronounced and tart flavor of apple cider vinegar.

For the Carrots
Nutrition Info: (Serving size: ½ cup without the optional ingredients) 31 calories, 0g total fat, 0g saturated fat, 122mg sodium, 7g carbs, 4g sugar, 2g fiber, 1g protein

For the Cucumbers
Nutrition Info: (Serving size: ½ cup without the optional ingredients) 7 calories, 0g total fat, 0g saturated fat, 71mg sodium, 1g carbs, 1g sugar, 0g fiber, 0g protein

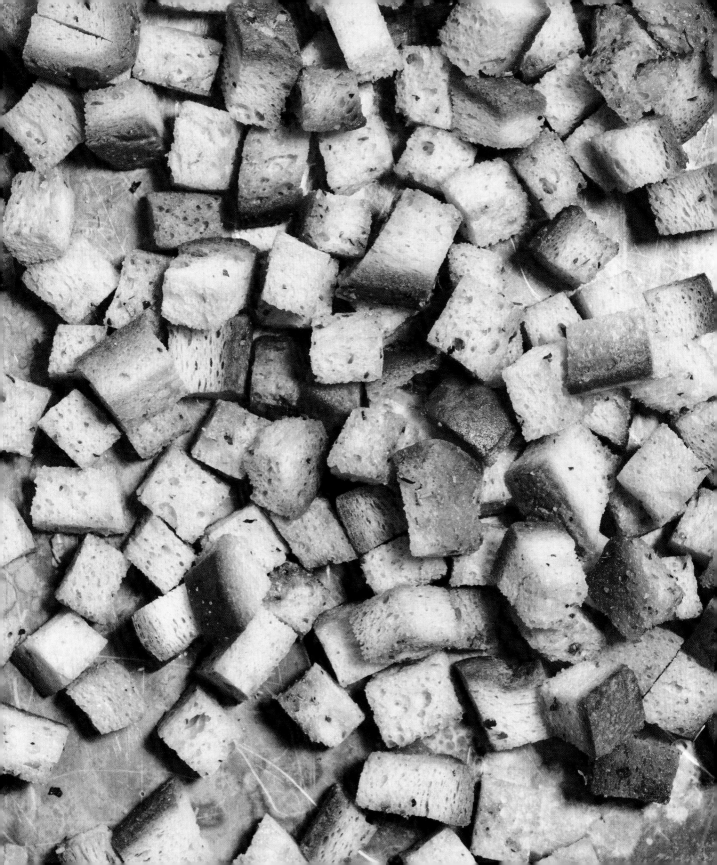

garlic-herb croutons

Prep Time: **10 minutes** | Cook Time: **25 minutes** | Total Time: **35 minutes, plus 15 minutes for cooling** | Makes **3½ cups (14 servings)**

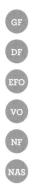

6 ounces gluten-free bread of choice, cut into ½ inch cubes (5 cups; see Tips)
2 tablespoons avocado oil or extra-virgin olive oil
1 teaspoon dried Italian seasoning
½ teaspoon garlic powder
¼ teaspoon fine salt

With just some leftover bread and a few pantry items, you can make your own croutons at home. These crunchy bites are sprinkled with garlic and Italian seasoning, perfect for serving on top of our Oven-Roasted Tomato Soup (page 193), Greek Chopped Salad (page 49), or Big Cobb Salad for Two (page 51). Making your own croutons is a good way to stretch your grocery bill, since you can use leftover bits of bread—any type works, even dinner rolls or buns.

Preheat the oven to 350°F. Line a rimmed baking sheet with parchment paper, if desired.

Place the bread cubes on the baking sheet. Drizzle with the avocado oil, then sprinkle with the Italian seasoning, garlic powder, and salt. Toss gently to combine, then spread in an even layer.

Bake for 22 to 25 minutes, stirring halfway through, or until the croutons are golden brown. (The denser the bread, the longer it will need to bake.) Remove from the oven and allow to cool before serving.

Store leftovers in an airtight container at room temperature for up to 1 week.

Tips from the Dietitians

For a vegan option that's also gluten-free, use an egg-free bread of your choice, such as Little Northern Bakehouse or BFree. If you don't need these croutons to be gluten-free, sourdough bread makes fantastic croutons!

Nutrition Info: (Serving size: ¼ cup) 56 calories, 3g fat, 0g saturated fat, 106mg sodium, 6g carbs, 0g sugar, 0g fiber, 0g protein

acknowledgments

to our team

JESSIE SHAFER, RDN: Thanks for having the courage to join the team in the midst of absolute chaos. Your words of encouragement and reminders that all the twelve-hour days to create the book on top of running the blog as usual and parenting would be absolutely worth it. We are so grateful for your willingness to just jump right in and put all your skills and knowledge to work. Thanks for being such a rock star!

ANA ANKENY: You have been with us since the beginning and truly a Jane-of-all-trades. Your endless support is appreciated beyond words. Thank you for taking a chance with us and agreeing to be our social media coordinator, recipe creator, gluten-free baking hotline, head of customer happiness, and, really, just our biggest cheerleader from the start. Thank you for being by our side through it all!

EMILY HASSING: To another OG, thank you for creating beautiful graphics to represent our brand in a way that's stunning, classy, and professional. You have an amazing talent of reading our minds when we send you a vague request for graphics, and you deliver exactly what we envision, even better. Your talents do not go unrecognized, and we appreciate you for not only that but even more for your endless support and for being one of our biggest fans from the beginning.

LISA GRUBKA, our agent: Thank you, Lisa, for hitting "send" on the email that started it all. Until that day we had talked about a book but always thought of it as a project for "someday." Well, that "someday" has finally come and we could not have done it without your support. Thank you for believing in us.

JUSTIN SCHWARTZ, our editor: Thank you for literally making this book possible, for guiding us through the process as first-time authors, for your inspiring creative direction, and your impeccable attention to detail. Without your support, this would still be a "someday" project and not a book we can hold in our hands and be truly proud of.

SUSAN CHOUNG: Thank you for your expert editing and recipe-writing skills. Having you function as a project manager in the manuscript creation process was a game-changer for keeping us on task and even ahead of schedule at times when deadlines were tight. Learning the art of recipe- and headnote-writing from you will serve us well for the rest of our careers as food bloggers and cookbook authors. We knew we were on the right track whenever we'd see a "LOL!" in the comments.

TO OUR PHOTO TEAM: Without you all, this book would be just words on pages. Spending a week in the studio creating the gorgeous images for this book was one of the highlights of our careers. You made the long hours and hard work worth it as you beautifully captured the essence of our work. Specifically, we'd like to shout out Eliesa Johnson, photographer, for bringing so much to the table and assembling a true dream team. Diana Scanlon, your food styling is out of this world. Everything you touch turns to visual gold. Jess Larson, we knew from the beginning that we wanted you to be part of this team. You know our brand better than anyone else, and we're so thankful you agreed to be our prop stylist. You knew exactly which props to use and helped make every recipe photo feel like "us." Thank you to our digital tech, Liz Bennett, for ensuring that every image was perfectly captured. To Madeline Fitzgerald, food stylist assistant extraordinaire, your cheery and bright attitude and kitchen prowess were the reason we could photograph so many images in a day. The food never stopped coming. Melissa Hesse, thank you for being willing to jump in wherever you were needed, for keeping us well-fed and caffeinated, and for bringing such positive energy and good vibes with you to the studio each day. And last but not least, thank you to Kristen Olson, owner of Studio Q. Your studio is a dream to work in, and your attention to detail, massive prop closet, and hospitality are unmatched. Thank you for sharing Nugget, your furry four-legged Vice President of Tastings with us. Morning full-body, tail-wagging greetings at the door and mid-day snuggles were just what we needed to keep us going.

TO OUR FELLOW DIETITIAN COMMUNITY: Your support does not go unrecognized. When you make one of our recipes or share with us that you have recommended our website, our recipes, or this cookbook with your clients, family members, or friends, it means the absolute world to us. Support from those in our profession is the biggest compliment of all and gives us all the feels. We strongly believe that together, the dietetics profession, can make this world a healthier place, and we can't thank you enough for linking arms with us to do just that.

to our families

FROM JESSICA: Thank you to my parents for instilling in me a solid work ethic and a can-do attitude. Thank you, Dad, for teaching me to cook at such an early age. As I teach my own children to cook, I am continually in awe of your patience. Teaching your children to cook is one of the greatest gifts you can give. Thank you, Mom, for being a super fan and one of the very first blog readers and email subscribers. Your support means the world to me.

Thank you to my husband, Dean, for being the greatest life and adventure partner I could have ever asked for and for holding down the fort, keeping our household running, and always being willing to pick up groceries, wash dishes, and eat more leftovers again.

To my daughters, Lily and Piper, you are my everything. You give me purpose in life beyond my career, and no one reminds me that life is too short to not enjoy the good things like you do. Thank you for challenging me and changing me in ways I never knew were possible.

FROM STACIE: Thank you to my parents for encouraging me to follow my dreams and for always being my biggest supporter both in the work that I do and really, in all areas of my life. Thank you for being a reliable taste tester with so many of the recipes found in this book. Also, a special nod to both of my grandmothers for teaching me how to bake and cook and kindling my love for all things food.

Thank you to my husband, Shane, for always being there for me. For your willingness to help with grocery shopping, kitchen clean-up after a long day of recipe testing, and for holding down the fort and occupying a determined little toddler so that I could test one more recipe. Your support day in and day out is a huge part of why I am here doing what I love.

Thank you to my children, Adeline and Jameson, for the endless amount of joy you bring to my heart and to every day. For being that constant reminder that there is a life to be lived outside of a career. You make my heart melt with every smile and giggle and I hope that my dedication to the work that I do instills in you the belief that you can do anything you put your minds and hearts to. Because you can.

index

Page numbers in italics refer to photos